Treating Bulimia in Adolescents

Treating Bulimia in Adolescents

A Family-Based Approach

DANIEL LE GRANGE
JAMES LOCK

THE GUILFORD PRESS
New York   London

© 2007 The Guilford Press
A Division of Guilford Publications, Inc.
72 Spring Street, New York, NY 10012
www.guilford.com

Printed in the United States of America

This book is printed on acid-free paper.

Last digit is print number: 9 8 7 6 5 4 3 2 1

Library of Congress Cataloging-in-Publication Data

Le Grange, Daniel.
  Treating bulimia in adolescents : a family-based approach / by Daniel le Grange
and James Lock.
    p. ; cm.
  Includes bibliographical references and index.
  ISBN-13: 978-1-59385-414-0 (hardcover : alk. paper)
  ISBN-10: 1-59385-414-5 (hardcover : alk. paper)
    1. Eating disorders in adolescence. 2. Bulimia—Patients—Family
relationships. 3. Family psychotherapy. 4. Parent and teenager. I. Lock,
James. II. Title.
  [DNLM: 1. Bulimia Nervosa—therapy. 2. Adolescent. 3. Family Therapy—
methods. WM 175 L433t 2007]
  RJ506.E18T744 2007
  616.85′2600835—dc22
                                                                      2006031305

For my late sister, Lizette—DLG

*For my family, without whose love and support
this work would not have been possible*—JL

About the Authors

Daniel le Grange and James Lock have been treating adolescents with eating disorders for a combined total of 30 years. They have devoted their careers to supporting parents and children with eating disorders in the treatment of these challenging illnesses. They have especially devoted considerable time over the past 5-plus years to learning more about bulimia nervosa in adolescents and how best to support families in their efforts to cope with the complexities and unknowns of this disorder. They are the coauthors, along with W. Stewart Agras and Christopher Dare, of the only evidence-based treatment manual for anorexia nervosa, *Treatment Manual for Anorexia Nervosa: A Family-Based Approach* (Guilford, 2001), and also wrote a book for parents, *Help Your Teenager Beat an Eating Disorder* (Guilford, 2005).

Daniel le Grange, PhD, is Associate Professor in the Department of Psychiatry, Section for Child and Adolescent Psychiatry, and Director of the Eating Disorders Program at the University of Chicago. He received his doctoral education at the Institute of Psychiatry, University of London, and trained at the Maudsley Hospital in London, where he was a member of the team that developed family-based treatment (the "Maudsley approach") for anorexia nervosa. Dr. Le Grange completed postdoctoral work at the Maudsley Hospital and the University of London as well as a fellowship at Stanford University School of Medicine. It is at Stanford that he first introduced the Maudsley approach to his colleagues in the United States. He is the author or coauthor of numerous research and clinical articles, books, book chapters, and abstracts. Most of his scholarly work is in the area of family-based treatment for adolescent eating disorders, including the first study of two outpatient family-based treatments for adolescents with anorexia nervosa. Dr. Le Grange was elected Fellow of the Academy for Eating Disorders in 2002 and has held several leadership positions at the Academy. He is a past recipient of a National Institute of Mental Health (NIMH) Career Development Award designed to investigate the relative efficacy of family-based treatment for adolescents with bulimia nervosa; the principal investigator at the Chicago site for a 5-year NIMH multisite study to investigate the efficacy of two psychosocial treatments for adolescents with anorexia nervosa; and an investigator on a 4-year NIMH multisite study of ecological momentary assessment of anorexia nervosa. Dr. Le Grange has lectured extensively in the United States, Canada, Europe, Australia, and South Africa.

James Lock, MD, PhD, is Professor of Child Psychiatry and Pediatrics in the Division of Child and Adolescent Psychiatry and Child Development, Department of Psychiatry and Behavioral Sciences, Stanford University School of Medicine, where he has taught since 1993. He is the director of the Eating Disorders Program in the Division of Child Psychiatry and psychiatric director of an inpatient eating disorder program for children and adolescents at Lucile Salter Packard Children's Hospital at Stanford. Dr. Lock trained in general psychiatry at UCLA Medical Center and in child psychiatry at the University of California, Davis, Medical Center. His major research and clinical interests are in psychotherapy research, especially in children and adolescents, and specifically for those with eating disorders. In addition, he is interested in the psychosexual development of children and adolescents and related risks for psychopathology. Dr. Lock has published over 150 articles, abstracts, and book chapters. He serves on the editorial boards of many scientific journals focused on psychotherapy and eating disorders related to child and adolescent mental health. He is a Fellow of the Academy for Eating Disorders and a member of the Eating Disorders Research Society. Dr. Lock is a past recipient of an NIMH Early Career Development Award; a current recipient of an NIMH Mid-Career Development award focused on developing and studying treatment of adolescent eating disorders; and the principal investigator at the Stanford site for an NIMH grant comparing developmentally tailored individual treatment to family-based treatment in adolescent anorexia nervosa. He has lectured widely in the United States, Europe, and Australia.

Acknowledgments

We would like to acknowledge the contributions of a number of our clinical colleagues in the development of this manual. We are grateful for the guidance provided to us by Bennett Leventhal (Chicago), Timothy Walsh (Columbia), Stewart Agras (Stanford), Michael Strober (UCLA), Hans Steiner (Stanford), Joel Yager (University of New Mexico), and Helena Kraemer (Stanford). The important work of our colleagues at the University of Chicago Hospitals has been fundamental in the initial development, piloting, and eventual empirical testing of this manual. Among these are Roslyn Binford, Maureen Dymek, Khytam Dawood, Marla Engelberg, Renee Hoste, and Chris Thurstone. Especially, we would like to thank the families who participated in the manualization process and who so generously allowed us to use their transcripts in this book. In addition, Dr. Le Grange was supported by a Career Development Award from the NIMH (K23 MH01923), and Dr. Lock was supported by a Mid-Career Award from the NIMH (K24 MH074467). Finally, and as always, we wish to thank our families for their support in our efforts with this project.

Preface

We wrote this book for clinicians who work with adolescents with bulimia nervosa. This manual is an adaptation of our work on adolescent anorexia nervosa (Lock, Le Grange, Agras, & Dare, 2001), an approach that derives from a family-based treatment (FBT) used first in controlled trials at the Maudsley Hospital in London, then manualized and subjected to larger controlled and uncontrolled trials at Stanford University and the University of Chicago.

Until now, our understanding of the treatment of adolescents with bulimia nervosa has been limited by the total absence of evidence-based treatment guidelines for this disorder in this age group. The present manual is designed to begin to address this gap in our knowledge and to provide clinical guidance about how to provide FBT for bulimia nervosa. More specifically, it directly results from experiences in adapting and practicing FBT with adolescents with bulimia nervosa in the first controlled trial in the United States, recently completed at the University of Chicago.

The overall strategies are similar to those outlined in our earlier book, *Treatment Manual for Anorexia Nervosa: A Family-Based Approach*. However, the differences in the symptoms of bulimia nervosa and in the personalities and families of adolescents with bulimia nervosa make the process and particulars of FBT distinct from that provided to patients with anorexia nervosa. Hence, this manual offers a new application of FBT for a related but distinctly clinical population. The form of family treatment described here utilizes parents as a resource to assist the adolescent with her recovery from bulimia nervosa. A key departure from FBT for adolescent anorexia nervosa is the fact that the adolescent with bulimia nervosa is enlisted to collaborate with her parents in their combined effort at her recovery. By contrast, in FBT for adolescent anorexia nervosa, the parents are asked to take control of weight restoration efforts and not to expect collaboration from their child until weight is restored and eating is normalized. For adolescents with bulimia nervosa, a more collaborative approach is possible in part because of the ego-dystonic nature of bulimic symptoms in most adolescents, a decided difference between these adolescents and their peers with anorexia nervosa, for whom symptoms are experienced as ego syntonic. In addition, helping the family to diminish the shame that accompanies adolescent bulimia is often an avenue for engendering increased collaboration between the adolescent and family members in FBT.

As was the case with our manual for adolescents with anorexia nervosa, our primary hope in developing this treatment manual for bulimia nervosa is to make FBT available in manualized format, so that more adolescents with this disorder can be given the opportunity to experience early symptomatic relief, recover from their illness, and resume adolescence unencumbered by an eating disorder.

We have worked as clinicians and researchers in academic medical settings for the past decade or so. Although we have worked in different parts of the world, our mutual interest in the treatment of adolescents with eating disorders has brought us together in our thinking about how best to undertake what we do on a daily basis in our respective practices. This mutuality has led to a rich and productive collaboration that is now approaching the decade mark. We started this collaboration in 1998 and jointly wrote our first book, *Treatment Manual for Anorexia Nervosa* (Lock et al., 2001), followed by a book for parents about eating disorders, *Help Your Teenager Beat an Eating Disorder* (Lock & Le Grange, 2005), and now this treatment manual for adolescent bulimia nervosa.

Contents

CHAPTER 1

Introduction and Background Information on Bulimia Nervosa

The Purpose of This Manual

Family work with adolescents who have bulimia nervosa (BN), though commonly provided in clinical settings, has little systematic empirical support, and therapists have few guidelines about how best to proceed with these interventions. BN is a disorder that primarily begins in middle and late adolescence and seems to bear some relation to difficulties associated with adolescent development. Therefore, approaches that take into account developmental issues associated with adolescence are probably most likely to succeed. In contrast to treatment for BN, family therapy to assist with adolescent anorexia nervosa (AN) is comparatively advanced. This manual is designed to address this gap and to provide clinical guidance on how to provide family therapy for BN. The form of family therapy described is specific in its utilization of parents and the family as a resource to assist the adolescent family member with BN. It is derived from the family-based treatment (FBT) for adolescent AN originally developed at the Maudsley Hospital and subsequently manualized for dissemination. As such, the manual's general interventions are identical in many cases and similar to those outlined in treating adolescent AN using FBT. However, the differences in the symptoms of BN, the personalities of adolescents with BN, and the families of adolescents with BN make the process and particulars of FBT substantively distinct from that provided to AN patients. Hence, this manual is at once derived from the FBT manual used for adolescent AN

1

while still offering a new application of the approach for a different population. It presents a treatment program that includes the details of specific
sessions and phases of therapy.

The manual is an adaptation of a recently published family-based
treatment manual for adolescent AN (Lock, Le Grange, Agras, & Dare,
2001). That treatment approach is derived from several controlled trials of
family treatment for AN (Dare, 1985; Eisler et al., 1997, 2000; Le Grange,
Eisler, Dare, & Russell, 1992; Russell, Szmukler, Dare, & Eisler, 1987) and
was subsequently studied at Stanford University (Lock, Agras, Bryson, &
Kraemer, 2005) and at the University of Chicago (Le Grange, Binford, &
Loeb, 2005).

The overall perspective of this therapeutic approach is to view the parents and other family members as resources to help adolescent patients
with BN. Parents, in particular, play key roles throughout the three phases
that comprise this treatment. It has long been advocated that the viewpoint
of parents should be taken into account when it comes to the treatment of
their child with an eating disorder (Lasègue, 1873). In fact, for most medical illnesses and many psychiatric ones, parents and families are usually
viewed as an asset. For a variety of reasons, though, families of adolescents
with eating disorders have been maligned, though with little evidence.
(Chapter 2 covers the full rationale for FBT.)

During the first phase of this treatment, parents are asked to challenge
and disrupt dysfunctional eating behaviors, including specifically binge eating, purging, and excessive dieting. To accomplish these parental interventions often requires reinvigorating parental roles related to controlling and
managing these behaviors. Empowering parents to take up these roles is a
main goal of this phase of family treatment. In addition, the therapy
focuses on supporting the disruption of these behaviors rather than on
other psychological or developmental issues. Often the therapist finds that
parents have not agreed on how to address the problem of their child's
bulimia, so considerable emphasis is placed on the need for parents (when
there are two) to agree on how to proceed. Nevertheless, the therapist
refrains from directing the family members toward specific solutions and
instead encourages them to work out for themselves the best way to challenge bulimic behaviors.

The second phase focuses on returning control of eating and weight-
related concerns back to the adolescent. This phase can begin only after
parents are confident that dysfunctional behaviors have abated. Practically
this means that eating behaviors have returned to normal, weight is steady,
and binge eating and purging have ceased. It is possible at this point to turn

to other family problems, insofar as they affect the adolescent shape and weight concerns and behaviors. Only in the third phase, when the adolescent herself* has demonstrated mastery over bulimic symptoms, do larger and more general adolescent and family issues come to the fore in treatment. Usually, this phase involves supporting the adolescent and family as the adolescent moves productively forward in her development. Specifically, this phase entails working toward increased personal autonomy for the adolescent, more appropriate family boundaries, and the need for the parents to reorganize their life together as their adolescent children become more independent.

The manual consists of 14 chapters. The first provides an introduction and overview of BN in adolescents. Chapter 2 provides an introduction to FBT for adolescents with BN and outlines in detail the therapy that will be the subject of the remaining chapters. Chapters 3–13 provide detailed instructions for how to conduct FBT for BN. Particular emphasis is devoted to the initial three sessions because these sessions set the tone and therapeutic style that are employed throughout the treatment. In these chapters, we describe therapeutic maneuvers undertaken by the therapist, their rationale, as well as illustrations of each.

In this introductory chapter we provide general background material on BN; the pertinent research literature, a profile of illness's presentation in adolescents, how it differs from adolescent AN, as well as treatment options and prognosis.

Overview of BN in Adolescents

Eating disorders are highly prevalent conditions that have a profound impact on the lives of adolescents and their families. BN is a disabling eating disorder that affects as many as 2% of young women. BN usually arises in adolescence, starting as young as 12 years of age, with peak onset at 18 years (Mitchell et al., 1987). Key features are binge eating accompanied by feelings of loss of control, guilt, and remorse. As in AN, there is a fear of fatness and repeated attempts to lose weight through dieting and/or compensatory purging behaviors (e.g., self-induced vomiting, laxative or diuretic abuse) (American Psychiatric Association, 1994; Russell, 1979).

---

*The feminine pronoun is used throughout this manual because most—but not all—patients with BN are female. However, this treatment approach is equally appropriate for male adolescents with BN.

BN is a major source of psychiatric morbidity and impairs several areas of functioning. Common comorbid psychiatric conditions include high rates of depression and anxiety, personality disorders, disturbances in social functioning, alcohol and drug abuse, and suicide attempts. Adolescents with BN experience significantly lower self-esteem than adolescents without an eating disorder (Crowther et al., 1985, 1986); in addition, adolescent patients with bulimia report significantly more suicidal ideation and suicide attempts than other adolescents (Franko et al., 2004; Hoberman & Garfinkel, 1990). There might be an association between sexual and physical abuse and binge and purge behavior among adolescents (Ackard et al., 2001; Waller, 1991), however, this issue has not been explored sufficiently in young patients. Beyond psychiatric morbidity, preoccupation with food and body weight can impair social, school, and work functioning.

Although BN is a psychiatric condition, it is also associated with significant medical complications, morbidity and mortality (Palla & Litt, 1988). As many as one quarter of patients may require hospitalization for medical reasons (Palmer & Guay, 1985; Fisher et al., 1995). Moreover, BN can be life threatening at times due to the physiological effects of recurrent binge eating and vomiting. Hypokalemia is common, and hypocalcemia, hypomagnesemia, hypophosphatemia, esophageal irritation and bleeding, Mallory–Weiss tears, gastric rupture, and large bowel abnormalities have all been noted (Schebendach & Nussbaum, 1992). The use of ipecac to induce vomiting can cause emetine cardiomyopathy, hepatic toxicity, or peripheral myopathy (Society for Adolescent Medicine, 1995). Body weight is usually within normal range, but dental caries, periodontal disease, and menstrual irregularities are common (25% of patients present with secondary amenorrhea, and 33% present with irregular menses). Potential medical instability in these patients, exacerbated by the fact that most tend to deny the severity of their conditions, causes a mortality risk.

Growth is a dynamic process in early adolescence, and severe nutritional deficits can occur in the absence of healthy and expected weight gain (Schebendach & Nussbaum, 1992). Early studies of dieting and binge-eating behaviors in community samples showed that 10–50% of adolescent girls and boys frequently engage in binge-eating behavior (Johnson et al., 2002; Jones et al., 2001; Stice et al., 1998, 1999; Whitaker et al., 1990). There is also evidence to suggest that disordered eating in males may be similar to that observed in females (Walsh & Wilson, 1997). BN may be as prevalent among non-Western and ethnic-minority females as it is among Caucasian adolescents (French et al., 1997; Stevens et al., 2003; Story et al.,

1995). BN is occurring with increasing frequency among adolescents and preadolescents. Applying stringent diagnostic criteria, studies have found that 2–5% of adolescent girls surveyed qualify for a diagnosis of BN (Walsh & Wilson, 1997). Several reports have described alarmingly high numbers of adolescents presenting with BN (Mitchell & Hatsukami, 1987; Stein, Chalhoub, & Hodes, 1998; Kent, Lacey, & McClusky, 1992; Russell et al., 1987). The relative frequency of premenarchal BN in children is particularly disconcerting (Maddocks et al., 1992). In contrast to adolescent AN, for which there is clear evidence that cases with early onset of illness have a better prognosis than those with late-onset illness (Steiner & Lock, 1998), the same is not true for BN. In a series of 32 BN cases with an age at onset of 15 years or younger, deliberate self-harm was more prevalent compared to later-onset cases. Nearly twice as many early-onset cases were overweight prior to illness when compared to typical, later-onset cases. Additionally, parental neglect was nearly twice as common in early-onset cases compared to typical-onset patients (Mitchell et al., 1991).

Clearly, BN is a highly prevalent and serious health concern that affects adolescents of both genders and across diverse ethnic groups. Although pertaining specifically to the treatment of adolescents with BN is limited, we review the available treatment approaches for adults with BN here.

Clinical Differences between AN and BN

Although AN and BN in adolescents share many clinical similarities (Le Grange, Loeb, Van Orman, & Gellar, 2004), the sometimes considerable differences between these two disorders need to be taken into account when FBT for BN is considered. There are specific diagnostic issues for which the therapist should map out a distinctive strategy for BN as opposed to AN:

1. *Comorbidity.* Perhaps the most prominent potential difference in clinical presentation between AN and BN is the presence of psychiatric comorbidities. It would be accurate to say that BN in adolescents covers a broader symptomatic front when compared to AN. The management of BN in adolescents may therefore be considerably more challenging, in that comorbid illnesses could conceivably derail the therapist from the primary task at hand. In AN, no comorbid condition other than acute suicidality

can trump self-starvation, making it more straightforward for the therapist in his/her attempt at "staying with" the eating disorder.

2. *Symptomatic emphasis*. Whereas AN is about the reduction of weight ostensibly for "health" reasons, BN is more about the overvaluation of shape. Moreover, the DSM draws a clear distinction between AN and BN; whereas the emphasis in AN is clearly on significant weight loss, BN focuses on binge-eating episodes followed by inappropriate compensatory behaviors, such as self-induced vomiting and laxative abuse.

3. *Family style*. Families of patients with BN are also perceived as presenting different relational styles from those of families of patients with AN. Whereas families of patients with AN tend to be more conflict avoidant and eager to maintain an impression of politeness, families of patients with BN often tend to be somewhat more disorganized and conflictive, inviting the therapist to establish some order.

4. *Pride versus shame*. BN is associated with considerable shame, and patients are reluctant to disclose their symptoms. For AN, on the other hand, shame is associated with eating, whereas patients often derive considerable pride in their symptoms. This difference may make change easier for BN; despite hiding symptoms, the shame associated with these symptoms may serve as a motivator for change.

There are also specific psychological aspects or characteristics for which the therapist should map out a distinctive strategy for BN as opposed to AN:

1. *Motivation on the part of the parents*. Young patients with eating disorders are seldom motivated for treatment, but with obvious signs of starvation in AN, it is probably easier for the parents to separate the illness from the patient and to be motivated to take charge of weight restoration. In BN, motivation is more mixed, and the therapist may have to work much harder to inform the parents about the secretive nature of the BN so that they can find a way to help their adolescent offspring who may not appear unwell.

2. *Independence*. Compared to the average patient with AN, young patients with bulimia often create the impression of having established a much greater degree of independence, even if this independence is often quite ambivalent. Whereas in AN the independence is usually self-willed, in BN it is more in reaction to others. In the end, neither the patient with anorexia nor the patient with bulimia is truly independent. The appearance

of greater independence can have obvious consequences for treatment, in that the parents may have come to accept the level of independence their daughter has established to the degree that it may be difficult to regroup to a position where they exert more control over her eating, and other freedoms, than they themselves would want to exert. Likewise, the adolescent with BN may not as readily accept her parents' perceived interference with her freedoms as many young patients with AN would. The parents' job is to help make the adolescent less anxious and to get back "on track" with adolescence. In other words, the parents are "repairing" their child; the adolescent with bulimia might still be regressed, albeit not as severely as the adolescent with anorexia.

3. *Psychological insight.* Some patients have insight into their dilemma whereas others do not recognize that they have a problem. The therapist will have much more of a challenge convincing the patient that her parents need to help her in her struggle with bulimia if she adamantly rejects the notion that she has a serious illness. However, in our experience, most adolescents with BN understand that they are unwell and are at least somewhat motivated to overcome their difficulties with eating (BN is experienced as more ego dystonic; see Chapter 3). On the other hand, adolescents with AN are mostly unwilling to entertain the thought that they are seriously ill—poses a denial that a particular dilemma for clinicians in helping these patients change their behaviors.

4. *Adolescent experimentation.* Adolescents with BN are more likely than their counterparts with AN to have experimented on a wider range of adolescent issues (e.g., romantic relationships, drugs). Not only may this complicate the therapist's efforts to keep the family focused on reestablishing healthy eating habits in the adolescent, but the parents may find it harder to intervene to the degree that the therapist may find desirable if they feel they have a relatively independent adolescent with many different experiences on their hands; someone whom they regard to be beyond their efforts at instruction or guidance.

5. *Peer pressure.* In keeping with the previous two issues, adolescents with BN are more connected to their peer group and may therefore feel more pressure to conform with the expectations of this group. Again, this may complicate the task of the therapist as well as that of the parents in finding a way in which they (the parents) can have a significant impact on the eating disorder of their adolescent in light of the expectations (e.g., for "perfect" bodies) of the peer group. However, the fact that the adolescent with AN is generally less connected with her

peer group and socially more isolated, makes treatment no less challenging, albeit for different reasons.

Treatment Approaches for Adolescent BN

Despite the availability of a large number of treatment studies for adult BN, none has specifically included or investigated adolescents with BN, that is, those ages 18 years or younger. Although AN and BN are distinct syndromes, considerable overlap in symptomatology is common. Therefore, treatments that have proved to be effective for adolescent patients with AN might also be beneficial for adolescent patients with BN. On the other hand, as noted, families with an offspring with AN may be different from those with offspring with BN, and these differences may have implications for the involvement of family members in therapy. Women with BN report more troubled childhood experiences than women with AN (Webster & Palmer, 2000). Our own studies have shown that there may be a greater likelihood of conflict or criticism in families with adolescent with BN compared to their counterparts with AN (Dare, Le Grange, Eisler, & Rutherford, 1994), but it is premature to talk about a "typical anorexic family" versus a "typical bulimic family." Notwithstanding, the secrecy of the bulimic behaviors, as opposed to the more obvious fragility of a starving teenager, and the general difficulty in engaging adolescents in therapy suggest that family intervention has an important place in both these disorders. From a developmental perspective, it is possible to argue that adolescent patients with BN or AN share similar challenges—for example, the negotiation of individuation, separation, and sexuality. Therefore, it is clinically feasible that adolescent patients with BN still living with their families of origin may benefit from FBT, albeit a therapy that accommodates differences between AN and BN in adolescents.

A discussion of family therapy for BN is incomplete without a brief reference to the Maudsley approach to family therapy for AN.

The Maudsley Approach and the Evolution of This Manual

The treatment of AN has been in the domain of family therapists for many years now (Dare & Eisler, 1997; Minuchin, Baker, Rosman, Liebman, Milman, & Todd, 1975; Selvini Palazzoli, 1974; Wynne, 1980), and family problems have long been identified as part of the presentation of eating disorders (Bliss & Branch, 1960; Bruch, 1973; Gull, 1874; Morgan & Russell, 1975). In fact, according to Dare and Eisler (1997), AN can been seen as paradigmatic for family therapy, much as hysteria was seen as such for psychoanalysis and phobias for behavior therapy. Minuchin and his colleagues at the Philadelphia Child Guidance Clinic (1975) as well as Selvini Palazzoli at the Milan Center (1974) observed specific characteristics in families with offspring with AN. They emphasized the overly close nature of family relationships, the blurring of intergenerational boundaries, and tendencies to avoid overt conflict. In the model of therapy advanced by Minuchin, the patient is seen as having developed a problem in response to various factors (e.g., familial, genetic, physiological, sociocultural). In this model, family intervention attempts to modify the problems within the family or, if necessary, remove the child from the family (Harper, 1983). In contrast, the Maudsley approach to family therapy does not apportion any blame; instead, every effort is made to resolve the eating disorder, in great part, by viewing the parents as a resource. The Maudsley approach for adolescents with AN uses many of the insights and techniques found in earlier family therapy schools (e.g., structural, Milan, strategic, narrative).

Although there are a variety of case series on many of these types of family interventions, only the Maudsley approach has been the subject of controlled trials. These trials demonstrate the relative benefit of family therapy for adolescent patients (i.e., 18 years and younger) with a duration of illness of less than 3 years (Eisler et al., 1997, 2000; Le Grange, Eisler, Dare, & Russell, 1992; Lock et al., 2005; Russell et al., 1987). The Maudsley group has been conducting controlled family therapy studies since the mid-1980s. The most prominent of these is that of Russell et al. (1987), which compares treatment outcomes in AN and BN. They demonstrated that, compared to older patients, younger patients with AN improved with family therapy more than with individual therapy. A 5-year follow-up of the original cohort confirmed the maintenance of the positive outcome for the young patients who received family therapy (Eisler et al., 1997). In a controlled pilot study, this group set out to explore the beneficial components of this family therapy, as well as demonstrating the viability of family treatment as an outpatient therapy (Le Grange, Eisler, Dare, & Russell, 1992). In a follow-up and larger study, they confirmed that family therapy for AN is a viable alternative to inpatient treatment, and that there is a relationship between family organization and treatment compliance and outcome (Eisler et al., 2000).

Family therapy has also been shown to be effective in controlled studies conducted by Robin and his group in Detroit. They compared a family therapy very similar to the Maudsley approach to individual therapy in 22 adolescents with AN and found that after 16 months, family therapy resulted in greater changes in body mass index, whereas both treatments demonstrated similar results in other measures (eating attitudes, body-shape concerns, and eating-related family conflicts) (Robin, Siegel, Koepke, Moye, & Tice, 1994). A 1-year follow-up of this cohort again demonstrated the superiority of family therapy in terms of greater weight gain and higher rates of resumption of menses when compared to individual therapy. Although individual therapy also proved effective, family therapy produced a faster return to health (Robin et al., 1999). It is clear from this handful of controlled studies that family therapy appears to be particularly helpful in the treatment of adolescents with AN.

Since these earlier studies, the Maudsley approach to the family treatment of adolescents with AN has been manualized (Lock et al., 2001) and applied with success in a recent large randomized trial (Lock et al., 2005). The present manual, although aligned closely with the AN manual, was carefully adapted to address the specific needs of adolescents with BN.

Family Therapy for BN

In contrast to adolescents with AN, there are few systematic accounts of family therapy for patients with BN. However, there are single-case descriptions of family therapy of adults with BN (Madanes, 1981; Roberto, 1986; Root, Fallon, & Friedrich, 1986; Wynne, 1980), and three studies of family therapy that give a clear account of this treatment (Russell et al., 1987; Schwartz, Barrett, & Saba, 1985). Findings from these studies were inconclusive. In the first randomized controlled trial of family therapy for adults with BN, Russell and his colleagues at the Maudsley Hospital found no benefit for either the family or the individual treatments. Swartz and his colleagues, on the other hand, found that 66% of 30 patients with BN improved after 33 sessions of structural family therapy over a period of 9 months. Neither of these studies specifically investigated at adolescent patients with BN. Early evidence that a psychological treatment may be effective with an adolescent population with BN comes from a preliminary report from the Maudsley group. This investigation of family therapy for adolescents with BN revealed encouraging results. The finding in a small cohort of eight adolescent patients with BN suggested that family therapy was helpful for this group of patients and their families (Dodge, Hodes, Eisler, & Dare, 1995). Inclusion of educational principles of the disorder and involvement of the parents in helping to stop the binge/purge cycle seemed to be successful. Most patients responded positively and showed significant changes in bulimic symptoms from the start of treatment to 1-year follow-up. These results should still be viewed with caution, however; this study described a small group of patients, follow-up was brief, and no control group was included.

Most relevant for the development of this manual, our own case study (Le Grange, Lock, & Dymek, 2003) as well as two large controlled trials of FBT for adolescents with BN that have recently been completed (see Le Grange & Schmidt, 2005) all show support for family-based treatment in this clinical population (see Chapter 2). Moreover, Eisler et al. (2000) and our own work (Lock & Le Grange, 2001) have demonstrated that the families of adolescents with AN binge/purge subtype respond well to parental attempts at curtailing bulimic symptoms.

As with many adolescent treatment paradigms, there are strong theoretical and clinical arguments for involving the family in treatment of adolescents with BN. Apart from any relevant family issues, heightened feelings of shame, guilt, and blame in the parents can reinforce the symptomatic behavior in the adolescent. In family therapy, information about the condition can be shared with the parents and the adolescent, and issues around meals and the impact of the eating disorder on family relationships can be addressed. Although sometimes not as severe as with patients with AN, adolescent patients with BN often exhibit a significant denial and minimization of the alarming nature of their bulimic symptoms that renders them incapable of appreciating the seriousness of their illness. This denial and minimization necessitate that the parents make sure that the adolescent receives adequate treatment. If the bulimic adolescent with bulimia is defined in the same manner as Robin, Siegel, Moye, Gilroy, Dennis, and Sikand (1999) conceptualized the teenager with anorexia—that is, "out of control" and "unable to take care of herself"—then the burden of providing that control and care must fall to parents. Parents of the adolescent with BN should be coached to work as a team in developing ways to restore healthy eating in their offspring. Therefore, FBT for adolescents with BN has considerable potential and should be investigated more systematically. More traditional approaches view the involvement of parents in the treatment of an adolescent at the cusp of establishing her autonomy as undesirable and inappropriate. Although individual treatment is preferable when parents present with significant psychopathology or hostility toward their adolescent, engaging them in the treatment of their offspring is almost always advantageous.

Outcomes for Patients with BN

A number of studies have followed patients with BN over the relative long term. Almost all of these studies followed patients who had received some treatment, and all of them focused on adults with BN. On the whole only about half the patients studied were considered recovered from BN (Fairburn, Cooper, Doll, Norman, & O'Connor, 2000; Fairburn & Cooper, 2003; Jager et al., 2004; Keel et al., 2000). There was evidence of increased comorbid psychiatric risk, particularly depression and substance abuse (Fichter & Quadflieg, 2004). Although overall mortality risk was not higher than expected in the general population, deaths have been known to occur (Fichter & Quadflieg, 2004; Herzog et al., 2000, Patton, 1988). Further, relapse was common in about one-third of the patients in several studies (Fairburn et al., 2000; Fairburn & Cooper, 2003; Herzog et al., 1999). Additionally, findings suggest that suicidal thoughts and behavior are common, with about a quarter of adults with BN reporting suicide attempts. One important predictor of increased suicide risk is younger age of onset of BN (Franko et al., 2004). The fate of adolescents with BN is largely unexamined in these studies, but it is reasonable assume that there may be an accumulated risk based on early onset and longer duration over time for adolescents with BN.

Introduction to This Treatment Approach

In this manual we present a specific treatment approach to BN in adolescents based on (1) our manual for adolescents with AN (Lock et al., 2001), (2) the recently completed trial for adolescents with BN at the University of Chicago (Le Grange et al., 2006), as well as (3) our clinical experience with this patient population over the past 5 years or so. By making this treatment available in a manual, we hope that practitioners who embrace this method will discover more about its appropriate clinical use. We recognize that no treatment works for every patient or family under all conditions.

Thus we believe that, other than in research studies where strict protocols are needed, the judgment of individual clinicians need apply. This need for clinical judgment is no less true for this treatment than any other approach. Therefore, although we have endeavored to be as precise and specific as possible in the forgoing discussion, we recognize and fully expect clinicians to modify certain aspects of treatment to fit the circumstances within which they find themselves practicing. At the same time, there are certain principles of treatment that would hold, we believe, in every instance. Among these principles are:

1. An agnostic view of the cause of the illness, which holds the family innocent from the perspective of treatment;
2. A commitment to the parents as competent agents for reestablishing healthy eating in their adolescent;
3. A view of the entire family as an important resource in recovery; and
4. A need to respect adolescent needs for control and autonomy in areas other than weight and food.

We also believe that the pacing of the therapy should follow the overall guideline of the phases of treatment. That is to say, the focus of the initial period of treatment must be on reestablishing healthy eating behaviors and weight control strategies under the direction of the parents; not until these issues have been resolved is it advisable to proceed to discuss more general family dynamics or adolescent issues. We have included an outline of therapeutic interventions for each phase of treatment (Table 2.1, Chapter 2, this volume). We hope that this outline will help therapists who are using the manual to keep track of where they are in the treatment process and to follow the steps as outlined.

The theoretical understanding or overall philosophy of the Maudsley approach is that the adolescent is embedded in the family, and that the parents' involvement in therapy is vitally important for ultimate success in treatment. For AN, and to a lesser degree for BN, the adolescent is seen as regressed. Therefore, parents should be involved in their offspring's treatment, while showing respect and regard for her point of view and experience. This treatment pays close attention to adolescent development and aims to guide parents toward assisting their adolescent with developmental tasks. To do so, fundamental work on other family conflicts or disagreements has to be deferred until the eating disorder behaviors have been eliminated. Normal adolescent development is seen as having been diverted by the presence of BN, varying, of course, in degree from patient to patient. The parents temporarily take the lead in helping their adolescent find ways to reduce the hold this disorder has over her life. Once successful in this task, the parents will return control over eating to their daughter and assist her in negotiating predictable adolescent developmental tasks.

The Maudsley approach differs from other treatments of adolescents in several key ways. First, as pointed out above, the adolescent is not viewed as being in control of her behavior; instead, the eating disorder is seen as controlling the adolescent. Provided there is no comorbid psychiatric condition, the adolescent is seen as not functioning in an optimal way and as possibly benefiting considerably from parental help. Second, the treatment aims to correct this position by giving the parents permission to involve themselves more actively in their adolescent's eating. Typically, parents feel that it is inappropriate to control their adolescent's life in this way and that they are to blame for the eating disorder, or the symptoms have frightened them to the extent that they are too afraid to act decisively. Third, the Maudsley approach strongly advocates that the therapist should primarily focus her/his attention on the task of addressing the eating disorder symptoms, especially in the early part of treatment. As opposed to Minuchin's approach, the Maudsley approach, tends to stay focused on the eating disorder for longer; that is, the therapist remains alert to the central therapeutic task, which is to keep the parents focused on reestablishing healthy eating in their adolescent so as to free her from the control of the eating disorder. The presence of comorbid psychiatric issues can, of course, derail the therapist as well as the family, because prioritizing the eating disorder in the presence of a severe mood disorder could be problematic. (See Chapter 2 for a more detailed discussion regarding comorbidity.)

Why Use a Manual?

Tension is sometimes experienced between the intuitive therapeutic relationship with a patient or family and the structure of a specific therapy described in a manual. This tension is, for the most part, a productive one. On the one hand, the particulars of each patient and family provide important information about the specific clinical situation at hand; on the other hand, the structured manual provides a general map with predictable guideposts that are relevant for many, if not all, patients and their families.

Some have argued that manuals are a "cookbook" for unimaginative therapists. These critics contend that patients are always, and in all ways, unique, and therefore their clinical needs cannot be anticipated by manuals. Further, they suggest that structured treatments rob the therapeutic situation of its soul by forcing both the therapist and patient into prefabricated theoretical structures and modes of interaction.

In contrast, defenders of manualized treatments argue that illnesses share common characteristics, modes of distorting thoughts, and reinforcing destructive behaviors. In this sense, a person with an illness is similar to any other with that illness. When an illness is diagnosed, the person with the illness joins the ranks of those similarly affected. For these practitioners, there is more appeal for an approach that anticipates the recovery process from an illness by providing both a general path as well as specific markers of progress. Following this line of debate, it is fair to say that there are benefits to both the therapist and the client when using a manual-based therapy. First, the structure, although flexible, ensures that the treatment procedures are sequenced in an optimal fashion and that all the components of therapy are adequately covered. Second, a manual keeps both the therapist and the client on track; without the structure of a manual it is easy to deviate from the central issue to issues that are not central to the treatment of BN in adolescents.

By writing this manual, our view of the usefulness of manuals is clear. However, few would argue that the best way to use a manual is to follow it to the letter in a lockstep fashion. Still, manuals are the only way, other than direct supervision, to provide therapists with information about treatments in a meaningful way. Effective treatments that remain available only in those few sites that develop them or become expert in their application are of limited value, because access is severely constrained by these limitations. Although a manual cannot anticipate every treatment problem or substitute for the unique relationships formed between therapist and patients and families, it can help to make use of the relationship in a focused way that is specifically designed to address the problem at hand.

Nowhere perhaps is the tension between individual needs and the benefits of a structured and specific intervention greater than in treating adolescents with eating disorders. In the case of BN, the developmental needs of a particular adolescent, in the context of the unique family context in which her illness arises, are set against the clear and compelling nature of the symptoms that link her to all other suffers of BN. In this manual we try not to disregard this tension, but rather to respect it. Therapists, in putting the manual to use, will find that it generally applies to the clinical situations they face with adolescents who have BN, but they will also find a need to use themselves as the means through which the treatment evolves. No manual can or should substitute for the basic respect, interest, and commitment implied in the therapeutic relationship. At the same time, few patients with the severe distortions in thoughts and behaviors that accompany BN would expect to recover on the basis of a therapeutic relationship alone. Finally, then, this manual is a tool for therapists, not the therapy itself.

Conclusions

In this chapter we have reviewed the etiology, clinical presentation, treatment, and prognosis of BN. We have reviewed these issues in part to provide general background information for the reader. However, we also wished to stress several important aspects of BN and its treatment that bear specifically on the approach used in this manual. The first is that BN is a disorder that primarily begins in middle and late adolescence and seems to bear some relation to difficulties associated with adolescent development. As such, approaches that take into account the developmental issues associated with adolescence are most likely to succeed. In addition, although treatment approaches for adolescent BN have not been studied, we have noted that adolescent AN family-based approaches may be superior to individual approaches. In addition, limited data show that this same approach may be helpful for adolescents with BN.

Emphasizing a family-based approach may seem counterintuitive to some clinicians who prioritize the adolescent's need for autonomy and self-control that is indeed an expected part of adolescent development. Instead, our approach emphasizes that adolescents with BN, because of the compelling nature of the thoughts and behaviors associated with the disorder, are out of control and need the help of their parents to "get back on track" so that the usual work of adolescent individuation can be resumed without the symptoms of the eating disorder. Thus, families are seen as an important resource for adolescents in their struggle to combat the illness and ultimately recover from BN. For most medical illnesses and many psychiatric ones, this view of the parents and families as an asset is the usual one, though for a variety of reasons, families of adolescents with eating disorders have been maligned, with little evidence.

The manualized therapy described in the following chapters takes these observations into account. That is, it is designed to specifically address the need for parents to assist the adolescent in reestablishing healthy eating behavior, and it also aims to support the developing adolescent in the context of her family.

In summary, although systematic evidence of any specific treatment approach for adolescent BN is lacking, the manualized treatment described in the following pages represents a reasonable approach. It is also an approach that is successful with adolescents with AN who binge eat and purge, yet is modified to address the differences between the two disorders. The treatment for adolescents with BN, as outlined in this manual, can be characterized by the following key components: (1) the use of the parents to help the adolescent reestablish healthy eating habits, and (2) a sustained focus on eating disorder symptoms until normalized; that is, while general adolescent and family issues are deferred until the eating disorder behavior is well under control. The advantages of this approach and a more thorough discussion of its merits are the subject of Chapter 2.

CHAPTER 2

Family-Based Treatment
for Adolescent Bulimia Nervosa

FBT for BN, as outlined in this manual, usually proceeds through three defined phases over a period of 6 months. Phase I usually lasts between 2 and 3 months, with sessions typically scheduled at weekly intervals. The spacing of sessions should be based on the patient's clinical progress. Toward Phase II, the therapist may schedule sessions every second to third week, and monthly sessions are advisable toward conclusion of treatment (Phase III). All sessions are 50–60 minutes in duration. In this manual we first describe the broad goals of each phase, followed by the specific steps that should be followed in order to achieve these goals.

The three phases of treatment are as follows.

Phase I: Reestablishing Healthy Eating (Sessions 1–10)

Treatment in Phase I is almost entirely focused on helping parents and the adolescent find a way to jointly devise effective strategies to confront the symptoms of BN and their destructive impact on the adolescent. At the outset, the therapist encourages united action from the parents to challenge and disrupt pathological eating and purging behaviors. Parents are encouraged to seek the collaboration of their adolescent in their efforts to confront the bulimia. This collaborative stance is one of the differentiating aspects of FBT for BN compared to AN; it is more feasible with adolescents with BN than with AN, in part, because of the relative ego-dystonic nature of BN compared to the highly ego-syntonic nature of AN. In our experience, most adolescents with BN experience their symptoms as undesirable, and although they are unable to refrain from engaging in binge eating and purging, many express the desire to be symptom free. Whereas many adolescents with BN remain highly ambivalent about the perceived benefits of their symptoms, most adolescents with AN view their symptoms as more desirable and will go to considerable length to prevent the efforts of others to alter the status quo. In order to help parents take action to help their child break the habitual binge/purge cycles that characterize BN, the therapist stresses that there is little evidence suggesting that parents cause BN. This information reduces parents' feelings of guilt and responsibility and frees them to take action. It also enables the therapist to express sympathy for both the parents' and patient's plight. The therapist directs discussions in such a way as to create and reinforce the parents' alliance around their efforts at reinforcing healthy eating in their offspring, on the one hand, while also aligning the patient with the sibling subsystem, on the other. The ego-dystonic effects of the bulimic symptoms complete the therapeutic picture by co-opting the patient's collusion with her parents' efforts to help her regain health eating patterns.

In a general sense, the stance of the therapist is to hold the family consistently and resolutely in positive regard, looking for opportunities for positive reinforcement and support by complimenting them as much as possible on the beneficial aspects of their parenting. At the same time it is important that the therapist show respect for the developmental status of the adolescent. In the case of BN, this almost always means helping to ameliorate the shame associated with binge-eating and purging behaviors and sympathizing with the plight the illness is creating for the adolescent. On the one hand, the therapist resolutely confronts the problematic behaviors, while, on the other, acknowledging the suffering and debilitating effects of BN. Further, the therapist acknowledges that encouraging parents to be so involved in their daughter's eating and weight behaviors is out of sync with what parents of teenagers would normally expect. The therapist clearly states that this degree of involvement by parents is temporary and only needed to help change the course of BN at the outset of treatment. This attitude might be conveyed in the following way:

"Everyone here appreciates the fact that you have managed to get on with your life as a young adult to a considerable degree, except for this area where bulimia seems to be in charge. The best way we can help you is if you and your parents can work out a way together that will help you eat in healthy ways again."

Sessions during Phase I are usually held weekly in order to ensure that early learning is quickly reinforced.

Phase II: Helping the Adolescent Eat on Her Own (Sessions 11–16)

Once the parents, with the participation of their daughter, have managed to normalize her eating pattern (i.e., no excessive dieting, binge eating, or purging), a change in the mood of the family is usually evident (i.e., relief after having taken charge of the eating disorder), and the family is ready to move onto the second phase of treatment. This phase aims to return control of problematic eating and weight-related behaviors to the adolescent, but under parental supervision. The goal is for the adolescent to master these areas with the support of her parents. This mastery becomes possible during Phase II because the parents and adolescent, working together in Phase I, have successfully broken the hold that excessive weight concern, inappropriate dieting strategies, binge eating, and purging have held on the teenager. In this context, family issues that relate to attitudes toward weight, dieting, and food can be brought forward in relation to BN and its emergence in the family. In this approach, family conflict, per se, is not necessarily viewed as causative in BN. If the adolescent is caught in the middle of the parents' marital strife, for instance, the therapist should address and attempt to resolve this issue, whether it presents itself in Phase I, II, or III. However, this treatment is not an attempt at marital therapy, and should this be required, the therapist ought to make an appropriate referral.

Sessions during Phase II are generally held every other week in order to encourage families to experience increased independence from the therapist's consultation.

Phase III: Adolescent Issues and Termination (Sessions 17–20)

Phase III is initiated when the patient's binge/purge symptoms have completely abated. The central theme here is the establishment of a healthy adolescent or young adult relationship with the parents, in which the illness does not constitute the basis of interaction. This goal entails, among others, working toward increased personal autonomy for the adolescent, setting more appropriate family boundaries, and the need for the parents to reorganize their life together after their children's prospective departure. Sessions during Phase III are generally held at a frequency of once per month.

Given the greater heterogeneity with which most cases of adolescent BN present in terms of family makeup, comorbidity, and developmental status, it seems conceivable that treatment sessions in each phase could vary from patient to patient much more so in BN than is usually the case for most adolescents with AN and their families. Therefore, the therapist should be prepared to implement this manual with the appropriate degree of flexibility but without sacrificing the integrity of the protocol. Flexibility is particularly required in Phase I if, in addition to the eating disorder, the patient presents with comorbidities that require immediate attention as well (e.g., significant substance abuse, severe depression). In these instances, the therapist will have to balance the attention paid to the eating disorder with the necessity to also address the comorbid problems (e.g., spend 60% on BN vs. 40% on comorbidities). In either case (i.e., with or without comorbidity) the therapist should work hard to put the parents in charge of managing the eating disorder at the onset of treatment.

Appropriate Candidates for This Therapy

The patients who are most appropriate for this type of therapy are 19 years of age and younger, diagnosed with BN and living at home with their families. We base this recommendation on the limited systematic evidence for FBT in AN and the clinical trials of FBT for BN. Defining *family* can be a contentious matter. However, for the purposes of FBT, a very practical definition applies: those family members who are living in the same household with the adolescent with BN. This may mean that a family session should include nonbiologically related household members or grandparents if they live in the home, whereas it may exclude parental figures who are not involved in the day-to-day care of the child with BN. We recommend this definition because parents and family member, to be of practical help in confronting symptoms of BN, need to be available routinely, especially at mealtimes. We take up the issues of single-parent families and divorced families later, but it is important to note here that these family configurations can be treated with FBT, though special allowances are usually needed to increase the likelihood of a good outcome.

Regardless of the specific family members, FBT requires a substantial commitment on the part of parents and siblings to attend therapy sessions. Parents must sometimes miss work, as they would for medical appointments for any serious illness; siblings often miss school or other activities. Families who are appropriate for this therapy must be prepared to make these sacrifices, though every effort is made to make therapy as convenient as possible and as short as possible. It is not possible to conduct FBT unless families attend sessions reasonably frequently (i.e., at least 3 sessions) per month at the onset of treatment. A family should be handled supportively when they fail to make scheduled appointments. It is important to not give up too soon, as the family represents a key resource to help the adolescent with BN.

Who Might Not Be Appropriate for FBT Using This Manual?

We should briefly note that FBT may not be helpful for other atypical food-related disorders in adolescents. Some of these disorders may have psychological and behavioral bases (e.g., conversion disorders, food phobias, psychotic delusions, obsessive–compulsive disorders), but there is no evidence that FBT would be helpful for these problems. In addition, FBT may not be helpful for adults with BN. By adulthood, there is considerable waning of parental influence and authority, so the leverage parents and other family member have to help challenge behaviors is much more circumscribed. Thus, the approach outlined here is most relevant for patients who are still dependent psychologically and materially on parents. There may be modifications of the approach that would be useful to young adults living at home, but systematic exploration of this adaptation is lacking, so it is not recommended that FBT, as outlined here, be used with adults with BN. In fact, when Russell et al. (1987) first studied the approach, adults with BN did not respond well to FBT and appeared to do better with individual therapy. However, college students, who are generally considered a high-risk group, could possibly benefit from this treatment approach if they still live with their families or if their families can reasonably be incorporated into treatment. This endeavor, though, remains highly experimental until more formal inquiry into its feasibility.

Who Should Use This Manual?

This manual is intended for use by qualified therapists who have experience in the assessment and treatment of eating disorders in adolescents. Therapists in training, under the guidance of experienced clinicians, may also use it. The treatment described should be conducted with appropriate consultation and involvement of professionals in pediatric medicine, nutrition, and child psychiatry. It is not intended as a self-help manual for either adolescents or their parents. A more appropriate source of help for parents and their adolescent is *Help Your Teenager Beat an Eating Disorder* (Lock & Le Grange, 2005).

Additional Professional Involvement

As is common with most therapy for children and adolescents, other professionals often are involved, either directly or indirectly, in treating the adolescent with BN. With AN, high degrees of medical monitoring often require pediatric expertise. Similarly, adolescents with BN, as noted above, may have medical difficulties. Of course, the degree of collegial (e.g., treatment team) and technical (e.g., video recording of sessions) support that the therapist requires will depend on his/her experience with families, in general, patients with eating disorders, and adolescents with BN, in particular. The availability and ease of access of this professional support will also depend on the setting in which the clinician operates. Few therapists, however, should aim to work completely without any support structures, because this treatment involves a complex therapeutic task, and it is relatively easy for the therapist to become caught up in family dynamics.

The therapist should coordinate regular contact with the consulting team members. These team contacts may be in the form of weekly face-to-face meetings, teleconferencing, or contact through e-mail or faxing. Of utmost importance is that the family therapist should be clear about leading the treatment philosophy while taking into consideration the available clinical data. Likewise, the team members should be familiar with the family therapist's philosophy and allow it to guide their contact with the patient.

Before the therapist's first meeting with the family, the patient will have undergone a physical examination. The results of this examination, along with a binge/purge log (described in Chapter 4 and included at the end of this chapter) and weight charts, are available to the therapist prior to meeting with the family. The therapist will weigh the patient during subsequent meetings and measure height if growth is predicted. Facilities to monitor weight, height, blood chemistry, and cardiac and endocrine status should be available or arrangements should be set up for routine medical examination and relevant laboratory tests. There are a variety of ways these arrangements can be accomplished, depending on the patient's medical status (e.g., regular orthostatic checks are advisable, as well as electrolyte screening in patients who purge frequently).

Many therapists will not have an institutional base to support their work. Many in private practice settings develop alternatives that are applicable and beneficial when doing FBT for adolescent BN. For example, it can be helpful, especially when first learning the treatment, to do so with a colleague. Pairing up can be advantageous in its yield of mutual therapeutic insight and support. In addition, because some family processes can involve the therapist in unproductive ways, working closely with a colleague can help prevent the therapist from losing track of her/his work and unintentionally rendering treatment less effective. Another alternative, or one that can be useful once therapists are working together, is to record sessions to be reviewed on a regular basis by an experienced colleague. If it is not possible to have a colleague join the treatment session, establish weekly supervision or consultation with a peer who would be available to review cases and provide the needed support and insights. Yet another alternative is to videotape or audiotape sessions for review with a colleague.

To prevent any miscommunication between the therapist and another clinician about the treatment procedures, it is best to establish a treatment relationship with just one or two pediatricians who can become familiar with how to best support FBT when they assess the patient. Still, because opportunities for misunderstanding remain common, regular meetings are recommended, especially when the therapist shares several patients with other clinicians. For clinicians in the United States, arranging for a regular pediatrician to support their work may be complicated by insurer patient–therapist purchasing agreements, which ordinarily do not allow for consolidation. In these cases, it is particularly important to provide the pediatrician with a good description of FBT and to keep educating him/her about the approach. Although this networking involves a good deal of work, it generally pays off in overall clarity and consistency of treatment; in short, patient and family are not confused by a barrage of mixed messages.

The therapist should take charge of organizing weekly team meetings or weekly telephone conferencing. In addition, the lead therapist should ensure that everyone involved in the family treatment shares all relevant patient charts.

Overview of the Therapy

In Table 2.1 we include an outline of the therapeutic interventions from Phases I to III. The purpose of the table is to help therapists see the pattern of the overall treatment as well as to serve as a tool with which they can track the progress of their cases.

Conclusion

In this manual we present a specific approach to the treatment of adolescents with BN. This treatment has empirical and clinical support mostly based on our own work at the University of Chicago and Stanford University. By making this treatment available in manual format, our hope is that other clinicians and researchers will follow the techniques and interventions outlined here.

There is no treatment that will work for every patient or family under all conditions. Therefore, in the implementation of the treatment described in this manual, the judgment of individual clinicians will apply. Although we have attempted to be as precise and specific as possible in our discussion of this approach, we realize and expect that clinicians will modify certain aspects of treatment to fit the unique issues with which a certain case may present and/or the circumstances within which they find themselves practicing.

In Chapter 3 we outline the necessary steps that comprise the initial assessment and preparation for the start of treatment, before moving on to a detailed account of the initial treatment session in Chapter 4.

TABLE 2.1. Outline of Therapeutic Goals and Interventions

Phase I: Reestablishing healthy eating (weekly Sessions 1–10)

Session 1: The first face-to-face meeting

There are three main goals for the first session:

- To engage the family in the therapy.
- To obtain a history of BN and how it is affecting the family.
- To obtain preliminary information about family functioning (i.e., coalitions, authority structure, conflicts).

In order to accomplish these main goals, the therapist undertakes the following therapeutic interventions:

1. Meet the patient, start binge/purge charts, and weigh the patient.
2. Meet the rest of the family in a sincere and warm manner.
3. Take a history that elicits from each family member how he/she has been impacted by the eating disorder.
4. Separate the illness from the patient.
5. Orchestrate an intense scene to convey the seriousness of the illness and the difficulty of recovery.
6. End the session.

Session 2: The family meal

There are four main goals for this session:

- To continue the assessment of the family structure and its likely impact on the ability of the parents to successfully reestablish healthy eating in their daughter.
- To provide an opportunity for the parents to experience success in reestablishing healthy eating and curtailing binge-eating and purging behaviors in their daughter.
- To provide the adolescent with the opportunity to convey to her parents the kinds of inner conflicts with which she struggles when she eats a "forbidden" food.
- To assess the family process specifically around eating.

In order to accomplish these goals, the therapist undertakes the following interventions during this session:

1. Examine binge/purge log and weigh the patient.
2. Take a history and observe the family patterns around food preparation, food serving, and family discussions about eating, especially as they relate to the patient.
3. Solicit the adolescent's cooperation in her recovery.
4. Help the parents assist their daughter in eating healthy amounts of food, including "forbidden" foods, and/or help the parents work out with their daughter how best to go about reestablishing healthy eating.
5. Facilitate supportive alignment between the patient and her siblings.
6. Prepare the family for the next session's meal and closing the session.
7. Conduct end-of-session review and close session.

Sessions 3–10: Remainder of Phase I

There are four goals for this part of treatment:

- Keep the treatment focused on the eating disorder and manage comorbidities separately.

(continued)

TABLE 2.1. *(cont.)*

- Help the parents take charge of reestablishing healthy eating habits.
- Guide parents to employ strategies that curtail binge eating and purging.
- Mobilize siblings to support the patient.

In order to accomplish these goals, the following interventions are appropriate to consider during the remainder of Phase I treatment:

1. Collect binge/purge logs and weigh patient at the beginning of each session.
2. Direct, redirect, and focus therapeutic discussion on food and eating behaviors and their management until food, eating, and weight behaviors and concerns are normalized.
3. Manage an acute problem (e.g., a comorbid issue) and then refocus on BN.
4. Discuss and support parents' efforts at reestablishing healthy eating.
5. Discuss, support, and help family members evaluate efforts of siblings to support the sibling with BN.
6. Continue to modify parental and sibling criticisms.
7. Continue to distinguish the patient and her interests from those of BN.
8. Close all sessions by recounting points of progress.

Phase II: Helping the adolescent eat independently (biweekly Sessions 11–16)

Phase II can be seen to consist of two parts. Part 1 deals with the transitioning of control over eating to the adolescent, and Part 2 identifies behaviors that might be associated with BN and general adolescent issues.

There are three major goals of Phase II treatment:

- To maintain parental management of eating disorder symptoms until patient shows evidence that she is able to eat in healthy ways and to do so independently.
- To return control of food and weight to the adolescent.
- To explore relationship between adolescent developmental issues and BN.

In order to achieve these goals, the therapist undertakes the following interventions:

1. Weigh patient at the beginning of each session and collect binge/purge logs.
2. Continue to support and assist parents in management of eating disorder symptoms until adolescent is able to eat well on her own without binge eating and purging.
3. Assist parents and adolescent in negotiating the return of control over eating to the adolescent.
4. Encourage family members to examine relationships between adolescent issues and the development of BN in their adolescent.
5. Continue to modify parental and sibling criticism of patient, especially in relation to the task of returning control of eating to patient.
6. Continue to assist siblings in supporting their ill sibling.
7. Continue to highlight differences between adolescent's own ideas and needs and those associated with BN.
8. Close sessions with positive support.

Although the treatment goals are the same for all sessions in Phase II, the emphasis of each session changes as the treatment moves toward the end of this phase. For example, Phase II sessions may start out very similar to those of Phase I, with healthy eating being the primary goal, but the emphasis will shift toward adolescent issues as the patient makes the transition from Phase II to Phase III.

(continued)

TABLE 2.1. *(cont.)*

Phase III: Adolescent developmental issues (monthly Sessions 17–20)

Depending on the tempo with which healthy eating behaviors can be restored, the therapist may find that more content and time can be spent in Phase III; that is, a transition to adolescent issues may occur well before Session 17.

There are three major goals for Phase III treatment:

- To establish that the adolescent–parent relationship is no longer defined by BN symptoms.
- To review adolescent developmental tasks with family.
- To terminate treatment.

In order to accomplish these goals, the therapist should undertake the following interventions:

1. Review adolescent issues with family and model problem solving of these types of issues.
2. Involve family in review of adolescent issues.
3. Delineate and explore adolescent themes.
4. Ask parents how much they are doing as a couple, separate from their children.
5. Prepare for challenges and issues that may arise in the future.
6. Terminate treatment.

PATIENT BINGE/PURGE LOG

Day	Binge	Purge
1.		
2.		
3.		
4.		
5.		
6.		
7.		

THERAPIST BINGE/PURGE CHARTS (page 1 of 2)

BINGES

	1	2	3	4	5	6	7	8	9	10	11	12	13	14	15	16	17	18	19	20
15																				
14																				
13																				
12																				
11																				
10																				
9																				
8																				
7																				
6																				
5																				
4																				
3																				
2																				
1																				
0																				

Session #

(cont.)

THERAPIST BINGE/PURGE CHARTS (page 2 of 2)

PURGES

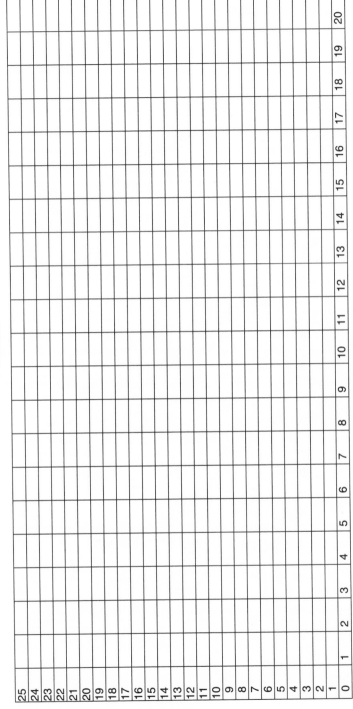

Session #

CHAPTER 3

Phase I

Initial Evaluation

In this chapter we briefly review an evaluation process for adolescents with BN. Initial evaluation, like that for many psychiatric disorders in this age group, is best conducted by separate interviews with the adolescent and the parents, followed by a medical evaluation and possibly the use of standardized assessment instruments. Next we describe the process that precedes the actual face-to-face therapy sessions. This process is a critical part of FBT for BN because it emphasizes the need for immediate communication of concern about the dilemma the patient and family are facing with BN. Setting up the treatment team and communication (telephonic and/or written) with the family detailing the high degree of seriousness and concern and the need for action to help the adolescent recover comprise this process.

Evaluation and Assessment of Adolescents with BN

Most often, adolescents with BN come to the attention of mental health professionals through a referral from a concerned pediatrician, parent, or school counselor. In rare instances the adolescent herself might contact a health professional to arrange for an assessment and treatment. At times family members may resist the idea that their child has an emotional problem or underestimate the hold that the eating disorder has over their adolescent; either stance fuels the avoidance of a referral to a mental health professional. Because dieting and weight concerns are central parts of

Western culture, in general, and of adolescent young women, in particular, it is important to distinguish between these typical and predictable concerns and those that become severe enough to warrant intervention. The standard thresholds for diagnosing BN are described in the DSM-IV (American Psychiatric Association, 1994). To summarize these criteria, BN is diagnosed when an individual engages in episodes of binge eating (i.e., consuming an amount of food that most people would regard as larger than normal, characterized by a sense of lack of control over the eating that occurs during such an episode), followed by inappropriate compensatory behavior/purging (most frequently, self-induced vomiting). To warrant a diagnosis, these episodes must occur at a frequency of at least two binges and purges per week for 3 consecutive months. Two subtypes of BN have been identified: purging and nonpurging. The purging type involves self-induced vomiting or an overuse of laxatives, diuretics, or enemas. The nonpurging type uses other inappropriate behavior to compensate for binge eating, such as fasting or excessive exercise.

Although some adolescents with BN tend to minimize their symptoms, in our experience, most seem to experience their BN as ego dystonic; that is, they are ashamed of their symptoms. Consequently, we have found most patients to be quite forthcoming with their concerns about binge eating and purging. Indeed, as a group, adolescents with BN are more forthcoming about their eating disorder symptoms than are most adolescents with AN. This openness is reflected in the differences in reports on symptoms, using standardized measures, between adolescents with AN and BN. In addition, as with any good adolescent mental health practice, it is imperative that the clinician also meet with parents or others who are likely to have important information about what has been happening with the adolescent around the eating disorder symptoms. The parents should be interviewed separately from their child because much information that parents would be reluctant to confide in front of their child can be obtained this way.

Interview with the Adolescent

In an evaluation interview with an adolescent with BN, it is important to convey support and warmth, while avoiding undue familiarity. Although an adolescent with AN might deny the existence of an eating disorder, the sufferer's emaciated state would usually be quite evident. In BN, though, most adolescents present with a healthy weight and do not necessarily look unwell. This benign presentation, coupled with the guilt and shame about symptoms as well as the secretive nature of BN, might present the therapist with a significant challenge in efforts to uncover the full extent of the adolescent's eating disorder. In order to gain the adolescent's trust, the interview can begin in a general way, with open-ended questions about her family, schoolwork, interests, and activities. Gradually, the interview should focus more on eating behaviors and problems. The therapist should look for initial triggers of the eating difficulties, which may be varied in nature. Commonly, these triggers include, among others, comments on weight (either on being overweight or a compliment on looking thinner), onset of menses, dating, family conflicts, increased pressures to achieve at school, a variety of athletic endeavors, and/or increased competition with peers. In addition, the therapist should carefully inquire into the manner in which weight concerns and concomitant binge-eating and purging behaviors started. Often the careful historian will discover that there has been a cascade of restricting activities, starting with ridding the diet of fats and sugars, then restricting proteins and meats, and finally restricting amounts. The therapist should inquire how this regimen of restriction might have caused bouts of overeating and carefully distinguish between a true binge (eating significantly more that the average person in a finite period) and a "subjective" binge (wherein the patient feels she has lost control, even though consuming only what most people would consider a normal amount of food). In addition, the therapist should ask how the adolescent has responded to these overeating episodes; that is, through inappropriate compensatory behaviors such as self-induced vomiting, driven exercise, laxative use, diuretic use or extreme restriction. Although the absence of menses is not a regular occurrence in BN, as it is in AN, the therapist should nevertheless inquire about the adolescent's menstrual status. In our practice, as many as 50% of all adolescents with BN in our program do have a menstrual abnormality. Because BN is often complicated by depression, borderline personality disorder, obsessive–compulsive disorder, and anxiety disorders, the interviewer should screen for these conditions as well. Throughout the interview, the therapist should be direct in the style of questioning and clear about his/her interest and concern.

Interview with Parents

It is best to have both parents present for the parent evaluation interview, especially when both adults are involved in the care of the adolescent. Not only does this step begin to involve both parents early in their daughter's treatment, it also provides important information about both the patient and the family that otherwise might be unavailable. Sometimes one of the parents is more involved with the patient and may not see things as clearly as a more distant parent. If one of the parents has been overly distant, the interview can serve as a way of "pulling her/him in" to help with the problem. Parents should also be asked about how they see the development of BN as occurring. When did they first perceive a problem? What have they tried to do to help? Do they see other kinds of problems, such as depression or anxiety, or other changes in behaviors? It is important to ask about their perception of their child's current eating pattern not only for assessment purposes, but also to begin a process of psychoeducation for the parents (and patient); it is quite possible that the parents are not aware of the full extent of their adolescent's illness, given the secretive nature of BN. The parents also should provide a general picture of their child's emotional and physical development as clues to temperamental variables, family problems, and family weight and shape concerns.

Other Aspects of an Initial Evaluation

MEDICAL AND NUTRITIONAL ASSESSMENT AND TREATMENT

In addition to the patient and family assessment, it is important to conduct a medical and nutritional assessment. These are important because they help to confirm the diagnosis and because the therapist needs to know the adolescent's medical status (e.g., hypokalemic) and how she will fare medically if her symptoms continue. A therapist should be careful to ensure that any patient with BN has adequate medical follow-up. As a rule, therapists should not take responsibility for this aspect of an evaluation or treatment; however, they should be aware of the kinds of assessments that a pediatrician or adolescent medicine specialist might conduct. A basic medical workup for an adolescent with BN would include the following: a complete physical to check for signs of malnutrition (e.g.,, dehydration and tooth erosion), as well as tests for liver, kidney, and thyroid functioning. These examinations help to assess the degree of illness, its chronicity, as well as to rule out other possible organic reasons for weight loss, including such conditions as diabetes, thyroid disease, or cancer (see Table 3.1). It is helpful for the therapist to understand the impact that bulimic symptoms might have on the patient's nutritional status, and consultation with a dietitian with expertise in eating disorders could be helpful in this regard. These trained professionals can also help clinicians determine the patient's current

TABLE 3.1. Medical Evaluation

Complete physical

Check for evidence of the following:

- Dehydration
- Orthostasis
- Hypokalemia
- Bradycardia
- Hypothermia

- Physical signs of purging (e.g., skin erosion on dorsal side of hands [Russell's sign])
- Esophageal tears
- Tooth erosion
- Weight and height

Laboratory tests

- Complete blood count
- Electrocardiogram (EKG)
- Electrolytes
- Blood urea nitrogen (BUN)

- Creatinine
- Thyroid studies
- Urine specific gravity

---

percent of ideal body weight, although this issue is seldom as pertinent in BN as it usually is in AN.

At times the clinician who is conducting an evaluation can become concerned about the immediate physical health of the adolescent. In fact, at any time during an evaluation or treatment, the need for an acute medical hospitalization may arise. The publication of medical treatment guidelines by the Society for Adolescent Medicine may lead to more consistent patterns of acute hospitalization for adolescents with eating disorders (Society for Adolescent Medicine, 1995). Although few adolescents with BN warrant acute hospitalization for their eating disorder, the medical guidelines suggested to assure patient safety used in this manual are based on these guidelines, as outlined in Table 3.2.

STANDARDIZED INSTRUMENTS

In addition to the usual clinical interviews, there are a number of standardized interviews and questionnaires available for use in the evaluation of children with eating disorders. The Eating Disorder Examination (EDE), a structured interview, is available in both an adult (Cooper & Fairburn, 1987) and child version (Lask & Bryant-Waugh, 1992). The standard form of the EDE appears helpful for most adolescents with BN, whereas for those under 12 years of age, the child version of the EDE is likely the best structured interview (REF) (Bryant-Waugh, Cooper, Taylor, & Lask, 1996).

Clinical self-reports are also available; for example, the Eating Disorder Inventory (EDI) has normative data down to age 14 years (Shore & Porter, 1990). Maloney, McGuire, and Daniels (1988) developed a child version of the Eating Attitudes Test (Ch-EAT), and Childress, Brewerton, Hodges, and Jarrell (1993) implemented the Kids Eating Disorders Survey (KEDS) for middle school children (Childress et al., 1993). Clinicians can make use of these structured interviews to illustrate treatment progress and highlight areas for further work. Most of these interviews take between 15 minutes and an hour to complete. At the same time, these structured interviews may be most helpful to the therapist in understanding the honesty, motivation, and particular symptoms of each patient. In our experience—and to our surprise—some adolescents with BN seem to be quite forthcoming about their bingeing and purging behaviors. As noted, this willingness to disclose is probably due, in part, to the more ego-dystonic nature of BN symptoms. Several of our patients have told us that they are ashamed to be engaging in these illness behaviors and wish there were a way to curtail or stop the urges to binge and purge. In Chapter 4 we more fully discuss the role of secrecy in BN, despite the relative candor in some cases, and introduce the therapist binge/purge charts to track these behaviors through treatment.

Conceptualizing the Case

At the conclusion of the evaluation, the therapist should be certain that the patient has a diagnosis of BN and should have identified any pertinent family issues that may bear on how FBT will be structured. As is the case with

TABLE 3.2. Admission Criteria for Acute Medical Hospitalization for BN among Adolescents

- Urine-specific gravity > 1.030 or < 1.010 g/ml
- Pulse rate < 50 beats/minute
- Orthostatic pulse change: Systolic > 10 mm Hg or pulse change > 35 beats/ minute
- Irregular pulse, QTc > 0.43 seconds
- Syncope
- Temperature < 36.3°C
- Abnormal electrolytes
- Physical examination consistent with dehydration
- Inability to curtail severe bingeing and purging

Note. Data from Lock, Le Grange, Agras, and Dare (2001).

adolescent AN, families may inadvertently reinforce the symptoms of BN. This is not to suggest the family caused the development of the disorder, but rather that certain family processes can interfere with resolving these symptoms. For example, some families consist of only the child and her parents. In FBT for BN, it is useful to use siblings to support the child with BN when her parents make decided efforts to disrupt her binge eating and purging. When FBT is applied in a family with an only child, the patient may feel unsupported. In these cases, the therapist has to do double duty in the sense that he/she must encourage the parents to take control of their daughter's symptoms while also being sensitive and supportive of the adolescent. This double duty is especially challenging at the outset of treatment, when there is little therapeutic rapport between the adolescent and the therapist. On the other hand, in these small families, there is an increased opportunity to focus on the adolescent because there are no siblings whose needs sometimes distract both the parents and the therapist. In these small families, the therapist must maintain an appropriate balance between the parents and the child that ensures that everyone feels supported.

A similar balance must be achieved in families where there is a single parent. In these families, the parental resource is half the usual, so the parent may come to view the therapist as an especially important resource. Of course, the therapist must be careful not to take up the partnership role. It is often possible to suggest that the parent find an additional adult ally (e.g., a grandparent, aunt, uncle) if appropriate and available. Nonetheless, the therapist should be prepared to face the reality that she/he will likely be needed more in single-parent than in two-parent families. The challenges to a single parent who is confronting the problematic behaviors of a child with BN are considerable. In this situation the therapist might expect that it will take longer for a single parent to take charge and manage these behaviors than it might for two parents. At the same time, though, care should be taken not to recruit siblings into quasi-parental roles because doing so would interfere with their ability to support their sister with BN. One advantage to a single-parent family is that there are no disagreements between parents about how to proceed.

Not all parents in two-parent households actually share parenting responsibilities; indeed, many two-parent families resemble single-parent families, at least at the outset. In such a case, the therapist has the challenge of finding a way to involve the uninvolved parent. There are a number of reasons that parents might not be involved with their families. One of the parents may be angry at, and frustrated with, the patient or self-involved with careers. Sometimes the role of parenting has been delegated to one parent, usually the mother, for practical reasons or for cultural reasons. Further, some parents who have removed themselves simply feel inadequate or uncertain about how to help their child. This is sometimes the case with fathers who incorrectly perceive BN as an illness that affects girls and women only. In order to bring the less involved or disengaged parent in as a resource, it is clearly important for the therapist to understand the reason for the distance. Therapeutic maneuvers designed to encourage the parental pair to work together do not change, but specific strategies will be needed to address whatever is preventing the distant parent from becoming engaged in the family. These strategies can be as simple as educating the parents about the illness to something as complex as recommending individual or couple therapy when severe individual psychopathology or marital discord are at the heart of the problem. Cases involving divorced parents and shared custody, where parents do not get along well but the adolescent divides her time between the two homes, also pose unique therapeutic challenges. The therapist must evaluate the particular needs and challenges on a case-by-case basis and help the parent(s) who is the more capable of supporting the adolescent in her attempts to reestablish healthy eating. Chapter 4 presents a full discussion of this situation.

It should be noted that sometimes a sibling may step in to take up a quasi-parental role, especially when one of the parents has removed him/ herself from taking care of the child with BN. It is problematic in FBT when a sibling takes over the role of parent because the *parents* ought to be doing the parenting. Further, as noted above, this also makes it impossible for the sibling to act in a supportive way toward the affected sibling. In these situations, the therapist identifies and directly confronts this problem and encourages the sibling to take on a more age-appropriate role.

Perhaps the most problematic, though not uncommon, situation occurs when the adolescent with BN herself is "running" the family—for example, in two-income families, when the adolescent shoulders responsibility for caring for younger sibs, and/or when a parent(s) has a problem such as substance abuse that creates parent–child role reversal. Often when this latter dynamic is the case, parents have tried to avoid confronting the adolescent about her behaviors out of fear that they will make matters worse, but this reluctance backfires and usually increases the impact of the illness on the family by disempowering the parents. In such cases it might be said that BN, rather than the adolescent herself, is "running the family."

FBT is designed to address the pattern of disaffection, avoidance, and inaction on the part of parents, but when these behaviors are entrenched, the therapist can expect to expend greater effort in inciting the parents to take action.

Styles of parenting vary from those that are quite lax to much more authoritarian approaches. In families with an unusually nonhierarchical structure, it sometimes seems that even at times of crisis no one is willing or able to take up a parental role. Without prior experience of exerting their authority, parents may seem overwhelmed by the problematic behaviors of BN. Often parents in these families have functioned more as "friends" or "collaborators" than as authority figures. Sometimes the child with BN has managed most personal decisions from early childhood. The task of FBT is an unusually tall order for these families because it requires, in the face of severe adversity, that the parents develop a new style of parenting that runs counter to their past models—and more than the usual conflict and difficulties should be expected.

The Therapist's Feelings toward the Family

With all these different family types, it should be expected that therapists themselves will experience a range of responses to them. For the sake of simplicity, we focus on two basic responses that can be problematic: liking a family too much or not liking it enough. In the early sessions in Phase I, liking a family too much might cause the therapist to try to decrease the necessary anxiety that is needed to generate motivation. It might make it difficult for the therapist to state the problems that BN has caused the family in direct and grave terms. In this sense, by liking the family too much the therapist enters the system that colludes with ignoring the illness and letting it continue unconfronted. On the other hand, disliking a family also causes problems. In these cases, the therapist's dislike interferes with the establishment of trust and can prevent the development of the collaborative relationship between the therapist and the family that is key to FBT. With intense dislike, the therapist may try to avoid the family and convey distance, which in turn leads the family to feel abandoned and unsupported. In addition, when a therapist dislikes a family, it is more likely that interventions will appear harsh and critical. When families feel judged and criticized by experts, their ability to take up the struggle against BN is severely compromised by the resulting feelings of inadequacy.

Although some might use the term *countertransference* to describe the strong feelings of like and dislike for certain families that therapists feel (and this might be correct in some cases), we wish to emphasize the importance of the therapist's feelings toward the patient and family. This stance is empathic, joining, and nonjudgmental, while still recognizing that there is a definite need for families to change in response to BN. If a therapist notes problems with maintaining this stance in her/himself, careful self-evaluation is needed and corrective action taken. As noted above, it can be helpful to track and understand the origin of unhelpful attitudes toward families by working in a team and consulting with others.

Comorbid Disorders

In addition to family dynamics, there are also factors intrinsic to the adolescent with BN that can complicate the use of FBT. Many adolescents with BN also have other psychiatric problems, particularly anxiety disorder, mood disorders, and incipient personality disorders that compound the problems of BN and make FBT more challenging to undertake. It should be noted that many anxious, depressed, and obsessive symptoms occur completely within the context of BN. Anxiety about weight and overeating and depressed feelings about failed dieting or insufficient weight loss are common with patients with BN, as are obsessive ruminations about these issues. It is important that the therapist clearly distinguish between those symptoms that are consistent with BN and those that suggest a separate comorbid illness. This is not an easy task because there is considerable overlap even when there are identifiable comorbid illnesses. Anxiety-related symptoms that are unrelated to shape and weight concerns and that predate the onset of bulimic symptoms suggest an underlying anxiety disorder. Similarly, a depression that is significant in intensity and duration and not associated with weight, shape, or eating supports a diagnosis of a mood disorder that is independent of the depressed affect commonly associated with BN. When these concomitant disorders are identified, the therapist must address these problems in addition to BN. In serious cases, such as severe depression with suicidal thoughts, the other disorder may take temporary precedence over the BN. On the other hand, many of the anxious and depressed symptoms that are a consequence of BN are usually effectively treated in the context of FBT and do not require an independent treatment regimen. Thus, the therapist would expect that by helping the parents master the task of reestablishing healthy eating in their adolescent, he/she may also provide them with the authority and ability to address or contain some of the patient's concomitant psychopathology (i.e., the side effects of the eating disorder). Still, when significant symptoms of depression or anxiety persist after the resolution of BN, the therapist should consider additional treatment for these symptoms, including pharmacological interventions.

Personality disorders are not technically diagnosed in children and adolescents, but by late adolescence consistent patterns of interpersonal interactions may be present. In adults, personality variables can have a role in predicting recovery and can therefore complicate treatments, including FBT (Casper, Hedeker, & McClough, 1992). Although the management of personality disorders is beyond the scope of this manual, the therapist will be required to consider a variety of personality types among the adolescent patients treated for BN. Some may be avoidant and anxious, others more histrionic and borderline, and a few may even have antisocial characteristics. It will be necessary for the therapist to adjust FBT in response to these personality variations.

Histrionic and borderline personality traits are relatively common in adolescent patients with BN. These adolescents may constantly test boundaries and display anxiety, self-destructiveness, affective lability. Needless to say, these types of behaviors are always challenging, but in combination with the medical problems and psychological preoccupations of BN, there is additional risk that these issues may derail therapy. In fact, it may be necessary at times to address these personality problems briefly in order to stay on track with FBT. Unfortunately, often such patients have families that are less organized or available to them, which may make family therapy more challenging.

In addition to these personality problems, some patients may be avoidant or overly anxious. Although not as common as histrionic and borderline personality traits, these two types occur commonly enough to comprise a predictable subgroup of adolescents with BN. Of particular note are social anxiety problems that complicate some adolescent patients with BN. In these cases, the development of BN appears to be partly a response to feelings of inadequacy about taking up social roles. The overemphasis on external indicators of attractiveness and the unusually high evaluation of self-worth in these terms suggest an underlying insecurity and poor self-esteem. Social anxiety results from wishing to avoid the experience of possible rejection or humiliation. FBT uses the family to support the testing of social roles and acceptability during the later phases of treatment, but at times these interventions are insufficient. In these situations, it may be necessary to provide additional care beyond FBT to address social anxieties that are unrelated to appearance.

Conclusion

A comprehensive evaluation that includes separate interviews with the adolescent and her parents is needed to ascertain the diagnosis of BN with confidence as well as to identify family factors that will shape how FBT is ultimately configured. In addition, this evaluation identifies other psychiatric problems, particularly anxiety and depressive disorders, and determines the degree of their relative independence from BN. In those cases when there are separate psychiatric disorders of sufficient seriousness to warrant treatment outside the parameter of FBT, the therapist needs to arrange for such treatment. Commonly, many anxious and depressed symptoms are concomitant with BN and can be expected to respond to interventions used in FBT. In the following chapter, we will provide a detailed account of the procedures involved in setting up as well as conducting the first face-to-face meeting with the family.

CHAPTER 4

Session 1

The First Face-to-Face Meeting with the Family

This first meeting with the family is crucial because it often sets the tone for the ensuing treatment. In scheduling this first meeting, the therapist makes an effort to impart to the parents the importance of meeting everyone who lives in the same household and that everyone has a role to play in understanding the illness and helping in the recovery. This message is followed by a detailed account of the goals and therapeutic maneuvers that are crucial to the successful conduct of this first meeting with the family. A troubleshooting section that addresses common questions and problems follows the treatment steps. Chapter 5 covers Session 1 in action with a transcript of a real therapy case.

Scheduling Session 1

Prior to meeting the family face-to-face, the therapist must begin the process of invigorating all family members to see themselves as resources in combating BN. To do accomplish this initial task, the therapist must do some preliminary work. It may seem unusual to make special mention of the initial telephone contacts. However, because this model is a time-limited treatment and success depends, to a large extent, on the therapist's ability to make a powerful connection with the family, and given the formidable task at hand, these initial telephone contacts take on a crucial role in facilitating the successful outcome of this process. It is therefore essential that the therapist (and not an assistant) sets up the first face-to-face meeting by contacting the family her/himself once a referral has been received.

From the outset of treatment, which commences with the initial telephone contacts, the therapist adopts a grave and concerned tone in order to convey the seriousness of the illness to the family. The tone and quality of the therapist's communications in this therapy are important for specific reasons (Haley, 1973; Madanes, 1981). The therapist conveys the seriousness of the daughter's illness to the family in a warm and portentous manner in order to raise their anxiety and concern and enable them to take on the difficult task the therapist is about to give them. It may be useful for the therapist, even at this early point, to acknowledge that the parents are demoralized and therefore skeptical of their capacity to do anything. Ensuring that the entire family is present for family therapy is a first step they can take to change these feelings. By setting up the initial family meeting, the therapist should achieve two aims with the phone contacts:

1. Establish that there is a crisis in the family and begin the process of defining and enhancing parental authority around management of the crisis.
2. Explain the context of treatment (i.e., treatment team and medical monitoring).

The therapist's first goal is to get every family member to attend at least the initial couple of treatment sessions. It is important to note the difference in this approach for BN compared to AN. Whereas in AN it is almost always helpful to have the entire family attend all meetings, the strategy for BN is more flexible in this regard. Meeting with all family members, at least initially, is essential, but it seems quite feasible to succeed with FBT for BN by working primarily with the adolescent and her parents further into treatment. The theoretical rationale for having all family members present from the outset is to aid the therapist in his/her assessment of the family, as well as to maximize the opportunity to help the family—the family plays a role in both the maintenance and the resolution of the eating disorder (Minuchin et al., 1975; Selvini Palazzoli, 1974; Eisler et al., 1997; Le Grange, Eisler, Dare, & Russell, 1992; Lock et al., 2005; Robin et al., 1999; Russell et al., 1987). If everyone in the family is not present, the therapist risks losing quite a bit of information regarding the family.

The therapist's second goal is to enhance parental authority even at this very early stage of treatment, to strengthen parents' resolve in making sure that all family members attend the treatment sessions and to begin to prepare them for the task of reestablishing healthy eating habits in their off-spring. The process of enhancing parental authority accords with Minuchin's suggestions about defining and clarifying hierarchical structures. From the perspective of structural therapists, strengthening parental authority, while aligning the patient with her sibling subsystem, enhances hierarchical definition and sets up healthy intergenerational boundaries. This clearer definition should enable the parents to embark on their task of reestablishing healthy eating in their daughter. Both these notions derive from the work of the Philadelphia Child Guidance Clinic (Minuchin et al., 1975; Selvini Palazzoli, 1974).

The therapist must make a decision beforehand whom to meet at the first face-to-face session, taking the context of treatment into account. Most often the therapist will use the initial telephone contacts to emphasize that there is a crisis in the family (but not of their making: that is, (1) their adolescent is overtaken by urges to overeat and then purges as a result of these binge-eating episodes; (2) they should respond to this crisis as a family; and (3) the therapist wants the help of all family members who share a household with the patient. Although this request that all those living in the same household should attend is straightforward in most instances, it may also require some firmness and tact. The therapist might say something like the following: "You are the people with the biggest investment of love and commitment to your daughter, so you are also the ones most likely to help the most with this problem." In response to alternative suggestions by family members, the therapist should insist that a whole-family consultation is the only way to address the grave family dilemma. This meeting should include the parents and their children, even adult children who may be in full-time employment. In addition, any extended family members living in the same household (e.g., a grandparent, uncle, or aunt) should be included in this meeting. If the grandparents are not living with the patient and her family but the patient spends a significant amount of time with them (e.g., the patient spends several hours a day with her grandparents after school and before her parents return from work), then the therapist may want to include these relatives in treatment as well.

In many cases parents are separated or divorced, which requires special arrangements. Initially the custodial parent and her/his household will have to be seen (the primary household). However, if the patient spends significant amounts of time with the remaining biological parent, then that parent and his/her household (the secondary household) will need to be incorporated in treatment at some later stage. The nonbiological parents/partners should not experience this arrangement as reconvening the former marriages, but rather as an attempt to develop cooperative parenting skills. These arrangements may seem confusing, but one way to proceed is for the therapist to determine after the initial assessment who is the primary family/household responsible for the task of reestablishing healthy eating habits. Such a decision should be made with the utmost sensitivity, and the therapist should take great pains to communicate to the families that the decision is based on their time and resources, and that it is not to be taken as a judgment of their ability.

There are a variety of common difficulties in setting up treatment. Should the parents continue to protest that it is impossible for everyone to attend, the therapist should reinforce appropriate parental authority in order to support the parents in convincing everyone in the household to attend. The therapist can begin by saying: "In my experience of this difficult problem, I have always found it best to meet all family members and learn how they view the difficulties, and it is important that you insist that everyone attends." That is, the therapist should impress upon the parents that they have a terrible crisis on their hands and that meeting all who live with the patient and getting their ideas about their daughter's/relative's illness is essential and extremely valuable. Stress to the parents that they have the ability and the need to convince their children and other household members that their sister/relative is gravely ill and that their opinions are valuable and very helpful in working out a treatment plan. The therapist might say something like the following: "Although it may seem inconvenient for other family members to attend family sessions, your other children will be interested in having their sister recover from BN. Besides, it's worth skipping school to attend, don't you think?"

A common question about FBT posed by many parents is: "Why doesn't this treatment focus first on the cause(s) of BN?" In response, it must be emphasized that when BN symptoms are very severe, the adolescent with BN is not in a position to explore or address the underlying issues. The patient and her family must wait until reasonable remission of bulimic symptoms has occurred. Hence, these issues that are addressed in Phases II and III of treatment.

Raising Parental Anxiety with Sympathy and Support

As mentioned, the first face-to-face meeting with the family is critical because it sets the tone for the initial phase of treatment. The therapist has already alluded to the importance of the first meeting through the initial telephone call(s) with the family. These contacts are designed to communicate the importance of everyone's presence and the seriousness of the therapy that the family is about to engage in.

There are three main goals for the first session:

- To engage the family in the therapy
- To obtain a history of bulimia and how it is affecting the family
- To obtain preliminary information about family functioning (i.e., coalitions, authority structure, conflicts).

In order to accomplish these main goals, the therapist undertakes the following therapeutic interventions (the "why" and "how" of each of these steps are discussed below):

1. Meet the patient, start a binge/purge log, and weigh the patient.
2. Meet the rest of the family in a sincere and warm manner.
3. Take a history that elicits from each family member how he/she has been impacted by the eating disorder.
4. Separate the illness from the patient.
5. Stress the seriousness of the illness and difficulty in recovery.
6. End the session.

The purpose of the first session is to raise parental anxiety and concern about the impact of BN on adolescent and adult development while, at the same time, providing sympathy and support. Another aim is to focus this anxiety on building a collaborative relationship between the adolescent and her parents so that effective interventions can be undertaken to combat the symptoms of BN. Every effort is made to reduce parental guilt as well as blame of the adolescent for the predicament that the illness of BN is creating for the entire family. It is especially critical to engage the patient in a sympathetic way and to emphasize that she *and* her parents' collaborative efforts are needed to reestablish healthy eating habits. The message the therapist is trying to convey is therefore a complex one that combines both a call for immediate changes in how the family is responding to BN because of the seriousness of the illness, while also emphasizing sympathy and a nonblaming stance toward the patient and family. In this context, the therapist should explicitly challenge any beliefs that the parents or the adolescent has caused the illness. This communication from the therapist is also referred to as a therapeutic bind (see Haley, 1973), wherein the patient and family are at once challenged to change their behaviors while also being warmly and appreciatively supported by the therapist.

Because of the secretive nature of BN, it is paramount that the therapist clearly describes the symptoms of BN *and* its medical and psychological consequences. In AN, the adolescent is obviously malnourished; in BN, however, the therapist has to raise parental anxiety around a constellation of symptoms (binge eating and purging) that they (the parents) might not have witnessed and that present in a healthy-looking normal-weight adolescent who is seemingly well adjusted. Conveying the seriousness of the situation can be a formidable task, and a very important one, if the parents are to be convinced to play an active role in helping their daughter overcome this illness. The therapist should succeed in raising the parents' anxiety so that they are now desperate for something to be done about their daughter's binge-eating and purging behaviors, and that *they* (the parents, in collaboration with their daughter) should do it. Although they may be apprehensive about taking on this task, the therapist's kindness and knowledge about how to get out of this dilemma encourages them to remain engaged and get on with the job at hand. It is this dichotomy in style—the therapeutic bind—that should help the family engage with the therapist in treatment. Put another way, the therapist aims to disorient family members by raising their anxiety, while being kind at the same time. This disorientation frees them from their usual patterns and allows them to take the therapist's lead and experiment with new patterns of behavior.

Meet the Patient, Start Binge/Purge Charts, and Weigh the Patient

Why

Meeting the patient, as in any other treatment, is obviously the first step toward forming a meaningful therapeutic relationship. Starting treatment by inquiring about binge-and-purge frequency over the past week and weighing the patient pose a real challenge to this first and essential therapeutic task. However, these first tasks do not just serve an instrumental goal; they also strengthen the relationship between therapist and patient by helping the patient through a potentially stressful process as the therapist communicates her/his understanding of this difficult process to the patient. The therapist is therefore able to use both the eating disorder symptoms (the actual binge/purge count) as well as the relational aspects that emerge from this process, in the family therapy sessions.

How

Prior to beginning the first family session, the therapist must first meet with the adolescent on her own for about 5 or more minutes to greet her, establish her binge/purge frequency for the past 7 days, and weigh her. More specifically, the therapist greets the patient and her family in the waiting area and asks the adolescent to accompany him/her to the office while the rest of the family remains in the waiting area. As the therapist and the patient walk to the therapist's office or weighing area, the therapist asks if the patient has any particular concerns or problems that should be discussed during the upcoming session.

Next the therapist asks the adolescent how many times she binged and purged in the past 7 days. The therapist also alerts the adolescent to the fact that she should keep her own record of these frequencies as the therapist will ask her this specific count at the outset of each ensuing session. The therapist will then chart the patient's verbal report on binge/purge logs that are kept in the therapist's file. Spending this time with the adolescent without the rest of her family allows the therapist to monitor her response to any change in her bulimic symptoms or her weight.

This process is repeated in future sessions and should become the expected and routine opportunity for the patient and the therapist to have a few minutes apart from the family as a whole to allow for communication and support for issues the adolescent may have difficulty bringing up without the support of the therapist. As treatment progresses, it is foreseeable that this initial 5-minute meeting is stretched to about 10 minutes or more.

At the conclusion of this brief meeting with the patient, the therapist will return to the waiting area to invite the rest of the family to join him/her and the patient in the office. The therapist shares the adolescent's verbal report of bulimic symptoms for the past 7 days at the start of each session with the parents, and this sharing helps set the tone of the session.

The therapist asks the parents to verify whether the adolescent's report reflects more or less of what they would have estimated. If the patient's account and that of her parents are in agreement, and the adolescent is doing well, then the tone of the session will be optimistic. If the patient and parents cannot agree, the therapist should take some time to help everyone reconcile these numbers. If there is lack of progress in terms of binge eating and purging, and/or weight is unstable, then the tone may well be more foreboding. Should the patient's symptoms remain unchanged or worsen, the therapist should use this information to reinvigorate the parents' efforts to help the adolescent reestablish healthy eating behaviors. In addition, the parents should be given a copy of the binge/purge charts at every session to serve as a visual reminder of their daughter's progress (or lack thereof) and their combined effort in reestablishing healthy eating habits. Unlike the case with AN, where the patient's weight is of paramount importance, the weight of a patient with BN should only be shared with the family when she is rapidly losing weight or if the therapist notes large and frequent fluctuations in weight, which are often a sign of excessive binge/purge behaviors.

Meet the Rest of the Family in a Sincere and Warm Manner

Why

Greeting the family presents the first opportunity for the therapist to begin the process of relating to the parents, patient, and other family members. The greeting is meant to convey both serious concern as well as warmth and understanding. The greeting must also suggest something of the therapist's expertise and experience as well as his/her openness to joining the family with their specific dilemmas about their daughter's eating disorder. Engaging patients with eating disorders and their families in treatment is often challenging, *and* the outcome of treatment is often affected by the degree to which the therapist succeeds in this task. When done effectively, the greeting has the potential to set the tone that ultimately allows trust to be developed in spite of the inherent demands of behavioral change that will ensue. Should the therapist fail in this task by not showing a sufficient sympathetic concern for the family's struggle, the family members might remove themselves quickly from the therapist's influence.

How

The physical aspect of greeting is often shaped by the individual therapist's style. Some therapists are naturally more physically warm and use touch or handshakes in greetings. Other therapists may prefer steady eye contact or nodding in the direction of family members as an alternative. When speaking with each family member, the therapist should focus clearly on the person who is speaking to ensure that he/she clearly perceives the therapist's earnest interest in his/her perspective. The process of greeting need not be a lengthy affair; rather it is the quality that is important. Although the therapist aims to make each family member feel comfortable, it should be clear from that the outset that in addition to comfort, some demands for attention and contribution to the tasks at hand will be required. This message is usually conveyed gently at first, through the interested greeting. When greeting each family member, the therapist may say something as simple as "*Tell me something about yourself, your interests, or activities,*" and then follow up with one or two brief clarifying questions such as "*What is it that intrigues you about X?*" "*How long have you been doing Y?*" The point is not to interview each family member at length so much as to demonstrate an even interest in getting to know each family member.

Take a History That Elicits How Each Family Member Has Been Impacted by the Eating Disorder

Why

In order to make efficient use of the first session, the therapist moves rather quickly along to take a history about how BN has been experienced by the family to date. The purpose of this history is to bring family members, including the patient, up to date on the problematic behaviors of BN. Each family member usually has something to contribute to this review, which provides the therapist with much relevant information but also brings the entire history of BN into the session as a common history for the family. Often this session is the first time that the family has discussed BN in this way. It is powerful to hear each family member's experience with, and concerns about, BN over the course of several months or years, depending on the case. The information collected here also provides the therapist with the "ammunition" needed to compel the family to action when orchestrating an intense scene later in the session.

How

This is a *focused* history for the purpose of raising parental concern about the BN. The therapist should let the family know that she/he is aware of other difficulties (i.e., depression or anxiety), but that the focus, for now, should be on the BN. The therapist uses a specific interviewing technique called circular questioning to engage and involve the whole family in this process. The therapist asks one family member to begin with his/her observations of how he/she remembers BN beginning. Once this person is finished, the therapist turns to the other family members and asks someone else to agree, disagree, or add to what has been said. A collective history is largely agreed upon by the time the interview is completed. Circular questioning also helps guard against domination of the session by a single family member or only a few members.

Separate the Illness from the Patient

Why

Separating the illness from the patient is a technique of externalization drawn from narrative family therapy. Its purpose is to permit parents to see that the adolescent is ill and in need of help rather than being oppositional, defiant, or willfully pursuing self-destruction through BN. Through externalization, the family diminishes blame of the teenager while also recognizing the need to take action against the symptoms of the illness as opposed to fighting with the affected child. In stressing that the patient has little control over her illness, the therapist tries to enable the parents to take drastic action against the *illness*, not their daughter. At the same time, this maneuver allows the adolescent to take some shelter from the shame she may feel about having developed BN. Moreover, separating the illness from the patient is an important way in which the therapist communicates support of the patient, who is now seen as having been overtaken by this illness. By repeatedly emphasizing that BN is not identical to the patient herself, the therapist can convey support for the developing adolescent and, at the same time, the strong conviction that BN is a problem for the patient. Research on expressed emotion has shown that parental criticism toward the patient contributes to early treatment dropout as well as poorer outcome in treatment (Le Grange, Eisler, Dare, & Russell, 1992; Szmukler, Eisler, Russell, & Dare, 1985). In addition, high levels of parental criticism and hostility toward the patient exacerbate the eating disorder symptoms and can have a negative impact on treatment outcome. Therefore, by modeling uncritical acceptance of the patient and her symptoms (i.e., showing the parents that most illness behavior is not within the patient's control), the therapist fosters a new understanding of the patient's behavior and reduces any parental (or sibling) criticism of her. It is helpful to specify that a noncritical attitude is not "normal" in most families but that it is therapeutically essential.

> "Sometimes parents have to do unusual things to improve their child's health."

It may be useful to provide an analogy of parents who have to do such "unusual things" as offering their organs for transplantation or providing an unusual amount of custodial care (e.g., cystic fibrosis).

In the process of separating the illness from the patient, there is often an opportunity to address the misplaced guilt parents feel for having caused the eating disorder. Sometimes they have read about BN and concluded that families cause the illness. Other times they may have tried to convince their daughter to eat or stop her from bingeing and/or purging, only to end up feeling ineffective and frustrated. They may have expressed anger and hostility toward their daughter. As is the case with AN, the perspective of FBT for BN is that families are not the cause of the illness; rather, the cause(s) of BN is unknown. More importantly, though, because families are seen as the major resource for helping the adolescent recover, any impediments to the family's active involvement, such as parental guilt, need to be addressed. Unlike anxiety, which we see as motivating parents to take action, guilt tends to cause hesitancy, self-doubt, and ineffectiveness. We therefore spend time in the first session (and in subsequent sessions when it resurfaces) directly addressing the issue of guilt to reduce its impact on parental action in taking charge of reestablishing healthy eating in their daughter. Separating the illness from the adolescent is therefore a helpful strategy in this regard.

How

The therapist should ask the patient to list all the things the illness has given her as well as taken away from her. As he/she listens to this list, the therapist must show as much warmth for the patient and as much distress and fear about the symptoms as possible, perhaps, saying:

"I am saddened that this terrible illness has interrupted your life to this degree, that it has taken your freedom away, and it has left you without much control over what you do."

It is vitally important for the therapist to show not only sympathy for the family but also an understanding of the patient. The therapist might continue:

"I know that you sometimes are more frightened of food and eating than of the thought of living with this illness for the rest of your life. The long-term consequences of the BN may seem a long way off, whereas food is right in front of you."

It is essential that the therapist attend to and modify any parental and sibling criticism of the patient. The therapist may point out:

"The symptoms don't belong to your daughter; rather, it is this terrible illness that has overtaken her and is determining almost all of her activities. For instance, it is BN that makes her hoard food or gets her to overeat or makes her behave in deceitful ways. In other words, it is the illness that gets your daughter to do all these things that you find so upsetting. The daughter you knew before this illness took over is not in charge of her behavior, and it is your job to strengthen your daughter once more."

Thus the therapist models sympathy and understanding of the patient to the parents, especially displaying a totally noncritical attitude toward the patient's symptoms and an understanding that it is the illness that has temporarily halted her development. To support this perspective, the therapist might say:

"I do not want you to feel that your spirit is broken. I want to help your parents restore your health, but not to give them control over anything else."

The therapist should also let the patient know that she/he understands that there may be parts of the illness, such as the patient's ability to restrict food intake, that the adolescent is proud of, whereas the binge eating and purging elicit shame. This strategy is key in maintaining engagement with the adolescent while attacking BN. Failure to achieve this separation can increase the patient's resistance to the treatment.

While going through the process of separating the illness from the patient, the therapist may find that family members respond to some of the patient's behaviors around food and comments about weight by being critical of her. It is not uncommon for a family member to say to the patient:

"What you do is disgusting! I can't understand how you can eat like that!"

or

"I don't know about this separating business. You're just trying to get her off the hook. She can stop this behavior if she wants to, but she lies to us. Every time she tells us that she's okay, I know she's just lying. She still binges and purges every day, and I can't trust her anymore."

Orchestrate an Intense Scene to Convey the Seriousness of the Illness and the Difficulty of Recovery

Why

In order to increase the motivation to take effective action to disrupt the hold that BN has on their child, the therapist must begin to focus parental anxiety on the problem. Usually, parental anxiety is present but unfocused and may be insufficiently high. By using the data collected during the family history-taking process and other clinically pertinent information, the therapist summarizes the story by highlighting the negative effects on the adolescent, her interactions with her family and peers, her schoolwork, and her emotional state. Note that this first "orchestration" is the beginning of a process that should be continued in the second treatment session. Anxiety is a useful motivator, whereas guilt and blame are not.

How

The therapist begins a relatively long monologue for the first time in the session; previously the patient and family members have been describing their experience of BN (see Chapter 5 for a full example). The therapist should view this monologue as a motivational speech designed to incite parental concern and to alert the family to the reality that BN needs to be challenged. The speech should neither blame the patient nor family. However, it should utilize, verbatim, as much as possible the examples of the problems noted and endorsed by the family members during their earlier interview. The therapist usually delivers this speech to maximum effect when these specific examples are incorporated. The emotional tone of the intervention is at once serious and warm, concerned and worried, with the goal of inspiring the family to see the need to challenge BN. The specific focus of the speech should be the patient's bulimic behaviors, the failed previous attempts at abstaining from bingeing and purging, the medical and emotional problems likely to occur if BN persists, and an emphasis that the family is the last resort for the patient. For example, if the patient has been hospitalized for the disorder, the therapist should alarm the family with the potential for rapid return to binge eating and purging. The inability of past health care professionals' efforts should be treated respectfully but held out as further evidence of the dire position in which family members find themselves. Regardless of the specifics of each patient and her family, the therapist should impress upon the parents:

"Although there are many opportunities for disagreement between members of a couple and between children and parents, when it comes to working out a plan about how to help your daughter defeat BN, you [speaking to the parents] cannot afford to disagree at all. Even a small disagreement between the two of you will make it easy for the eating disorder to remain central to your daughter's life and defeat her."

Upon gathering information from family members about how they experience the illness, the therapist reflects and amplifies what they have told her about the effects of BN in a way that stresses the seriousness of the illness. In order to be successful, the therapist should be genuine and purposeful when expressing the horror, despair, panic, and hopelessness of the family up to this point. Often the therapist finds it helpful to integrate the very real medical and psychological problems common to BN into this recitation. Also, the therapist must work hard not to accept the "BN façade" that so successfully hides the eating disorder from view. That is, the deceitful nature of the illness, coupled with a healthy-looking adolescent, can easily convince even an experienced therapist that the symptoms have largely dissipated and that the adolescent is happy and well adjusted within her family and with her peers. The therapist must try to raise the family's energy levels because default settings related to habit, family structure, and patient resistance may inhibit the parents' ability to take charge of the process of reestablishing healthy eating in their daughter.

End the Session

The therapist ends the session with great sympathy and sorrow as well as a sense of optimism that the parents will be able to work out a way to save their daughter's life. Thus, the therapist leaves the family with a sense of responsibility to take on this awesome task of reestablishing healthy eating habits in their daughter.

End-of-Session Review

As should be the case at the end of each treatment session, the lead therapist should communicate with therapy and consultation team members and review the following questions.

Session 1 Troubleshooting

• *What if some family members fail to show up for the first session?* The therapist's response will, in part, depend on how closely he/she adheres to a purist view of family therapy—that is, subscribing only to conjoint family therapy or to the view that a family consists of several subsystems that can be seen separately in treatment. Some therapists make it very clear to the family from the outset that they only work with the family when all members are present and may even decline to interview an "incomplete" family. We would, however, advocate a more accommodating view. The advantage of going ahead with the meeting despite the absence of some family members is that the therapist indicates the urgency to attend to the illness without delay. Given the serious nature of the illness, it may be unadvisable to let the family return home "empty-handed," so the therapist may choose to interview the patient and all family members who are present for the first session. The therapist can then use this first face-to-face session to stress the importance of meeting every member of the patient's household and encourage the present members to cajole the absent member(s) to attend the next family meeting.

The risk in going ahead with meeting an incomplete family is twofold. First, the therapist is somewhat hampered in his/her efforts to engage all family members in addressing the patient's eating disorder symptoms, in that he/she does not get the opportunity to see the family as a whole and can only make inferences regarding interaction patterns between the present and absent members. Second, starting therapy without everyone present may reinforce for those present, as well as for the absentees, that treatment can continue without the absent family members. Having said all this though, in practice, considerable flexibility on the part of the therapist should allow for a more accommodating stance insofar as who comprises the core family members and who can successfully help the adolescent address her bulimic symptoms.

• *What if the patient does not want her family to know about her binge eating and purging or her weight?* Many patients resist the idea of their families knowing the extent of their bingeing and purging or have knowledge of their weight mostly out of embarrassment and shame, but also to prevent parents from intervening. Consequently, the therapist may feel trapped between showing respect for the developing adolescent's autonomy, on the one hand, and getting on with treatment on the other. One way to handle this dilemma is to address both parents and patient. Turning to the parents, the therapist may say:

> "Although the patient is a young adult in many respects, when it comes to eating and weight, we all need to have the facts about the eating disorder on the table. It is very important for you as parents to find a way to help her out in this regard, until she can maintain a healthy weight and remain free of binge eating and purging. To be successful at this task, it will be imperative that we monitor her weight from time to time, but especially monitor the bulimic behaviors together at each session."

Turning to the patient, the therapist may say:

> "I know this is awful for you, and you must be upset with all of us for telling you what to do. I am sorry for that, but while you are so terribly caught up in this eating disorder, it would be dangerous for me to listen to your bulimia speaking, because this illness will not allow you to get healthy, and we cannot let that happen."

This personification of BN is a method of externalizing the illness, that is, separating the patient from the illness, as noted, and is demonstrated more clearly in the transcribed case in the next chapter.

• *What if the patient expresses a wish not to be weighed?* Unlike AN, the patient with BN seldom refuses to be weighed. When it does occur, the therapist should show his/her understanding of the patient's reluctance.

However, because weight stability (for most patients) and abstinence from binge eating and purging are the essence of the treatment, especially during Phase I, the therapist takes a firm but gentle stance that there is no way forward unless weight status is checked routinely by the therapist, but especially at the start of treatment. When this view is stated with conviction and compassion and without apology, very few patients resist being weighed. If the patient's weight is too high, the therapist would reassure her that regular healthy eating will most likely result in some weight loss and a move closer to a healthy level for age and height. If a patient's weight is too low, then obviously the therapist would want to comment on the need to gain some weight and keep a close check on how the patient is progressing on this score.

- *What if problems other than the BN come to light?* Unlike the case in AN, where nothing can trump self-starvation (with the exception of acute suicidality), a focus on BN could be derailed relatively easily by a variety of comorbid psychiatric conditions. The therapist should attempt to retain the primary focus on the BN while also attending to the concomitant depression, substance abuse, or anxiety. Although spending the bulk of the time addressing the eating disorder, the therapist should assess the severity of the comorbid condition to determine whether this condition can also be managed in the context of FBT, or whether it warrants treatment outside the confines of this manual (e.g., by another team member, such as a child and adolescent psychiatrist). Preferably, a team member can manage this comorbid condition while the primary clinician remains focused on the resolution of the eating disorder.

- *What if the patient does not comply with the request to keep a weekly binge/purge log?* Such refusal is quite likely and will pose considerable problems for the therapist. Due to the secretive nature of BN as well as the patient's shame about her symptoms, great reluctance to share details of these behaviors with the therapist is highly likely. The therapist should take great pains to help the patient realize that her behavior, albeit very worrisome, is understood by the therapist and that she/he realizes that the behavior is outside the patient's control. However, it is only with knowledge about the severity or intensity of the symptoms that the therapist will be able to fully understand the illness and assist the patient and her parents to find a way of overcoming the BN.

- *What if the patient refuses parental support?* For the patient to refuse parental support is not an option, although the collaborative nature of the parents' approach to treatment should, in practice, counteract most adolescents' efforts at precluding their parents' support. The parents have to set up a meal regimen at home during which eating a healthy meal promptly occurs—the expectation for this to occur is relentlessly powerful. In other words, the culture that is created by the parents is that there is no alternative to eating/compliance and subsequent supervision in order to prevent purging. This is similar to the culture/meal regimen that occurs in a well-functioning dedicated eating disorders service. If the parents succeed in closing all the loopholes for bulimic behaviors, it would be impossible for the adolescent to be able to refuse support. Setting up such a regimen requires time and patience, and the therapist must review exactly how the parents and their adolescent have gone about setting up this regimen every week. In order to help the patient to understand why her parents are setting up such a regimen, the therapist may say:

"Your parents will want to be able to reassure you and themselves that, should you become even more unwell because of the bulimia, they have tried their best to help you battle this illness."

• *What if the siblings are resistant to help their sister?* Many siblings do not show obvious signs of concern with their sister's illness, in part because they might not know about its presence or because they might not fully appreciate the medical and psychiatric consequences of the eating disorder. In addition, they may also feel discouraged by previous failed attempts to help their sibling recover, or they may in fact be jealous of all the attention being focused on the patient because of her illness. In very rare instances may we find a sibling who starts developing a problem and acts out for attention. Some siblings may appear to have given up on their ill sister and are somewhat resistant in helping any further. As may be the case with the parents, it is imperative that the therapist raise the siblings' level of concern for their sister and tell them how crucial their behavior will be in helping their sister. The therapist may say:

"Brothers and sisters become more and more important as you grow older. You can't afford to lose one."

Insisting that their presence at every treatment session is helpful, while making sure that information is gathered from each and every member during the sessions, will help to convince the siblings that their presence in the session and assistance at home indeed make a difference to their sister's well-being. It is the principal job of the siblings to support their ill sister through this period, not to direct their efforts toward regulating her eating, because this is the task of the parents in collaboration with their ill off-spring.

• *What if the therapist becomes emotionally involved with the family?* Making an accurate assessment of the family is sometimes compromised by the way in which the therapist becomes absorbed into the family. This absorption may occur because our social training often leads us to accommodate ourselves to the family pattern, adjusting our role and style to fit that of the family. Because this absorption is professionally potentially hazardous—for example, the risk of unconsciously fitting into the family patterns in a way that renders the family ineffective in overcoming the patient's eating disorder—a cotherapist, supervising peer, or observing team is important. The role of the supervisor is to modify and develop the therapist's direct response to the patient's family.

• *What if the patient becomes too ill to be treated outside the hospital?* If the therapist experiences difficulty in getting the parents to reestablish healthy eating in their daughter and prevent her from binge eating and purging, in some instances (albeit relatively rare in BN) the patient may become too ill to be treated outside the hospital. The therapist will have to use his/her best judgment here to determine at what juncture he/she will recommend that the patient should be hospitalized (e.g., a medical juncture, when the patient becomes hypokalemic, or a psychiatric one when the patient is otherwise medically stable but unable to interrupt the binge/purge cycle). This hospitalization, of course, would be an unfortunate turn of events and might complicate treatment on several levels. First, obtaining a bed in a specialist eating disorders inpatient unit may prove quite a challenge. Second, the parents may experience a move to an inpatient facility as a further failure on their part, and the patient may become more entrenched in her eating disorder. Third, once the patient is discharged from the hospital, reengaging the family in an effort to mobilize them to make another attempt at this difficult task may prove unsuccessful. Clearly, the therapist should work hard to prevent this scenario from unfolding. The therapist may find the criteria for inpatient treatment included in Chapter 2 helpful.

After a patient is hospitalized, it is still possible to continue the family-based approach used in this manual. However, FBT in the hospital will be limited in scope. Because the family is unlikely to be able to participate in their child's day-to-day treatment in an inpatient setting, family work should emphasize the seriousness of the medical problems their child is experiencing and the need for action on the parents' part to turn this situation around once the adolescent is discharged. The occasion of the hospitalization may serve as needed evidence that the eating problem is severe and requires that the parents devote themselves to the effort of overcoming the disorder. In short, hospitalization can serve as a new crisis to encourage aggressive action by the parents. On the other hand, as noted a hospital admission may be experienced as a failure on the part of the family and the therapist. Such a perspective is not helpful and should be avoided. Instead, focus should be maintained on the need for the parents to pick up the process to reestablish healthy eating after their child is discharged. Continuing to support the parents in developing their sense of empowerment may be difficult in a hospital setting, but should be undertaken.

This chapter provides a detailed account of the therapeutic steps the therapist should take in order to bring Session 1 to a successful resolution. In Chapter 5 we provide an example of a real case and the challenges the therapist had to negotiate in the process of following the steps as outlined in this chapter.

CHAPTER 5

Session I in Action

This chapter provides a real-life example of Session 1, beginning with a brief background note about the patient and her family (identifying details altered to protect the family's identity). The session is divided into major parts by the intervention. In addition, explanatory notes are added as the session unfolds to highlight the specific aims the therapist has in mind.

By way of a review, the main goals for the first session are:

• To engage the family in the therapy.
• To obtain a history of BN and how it is affecting the family.
• To obtain preliminary information about family functioning (i.e., coalitions, authority structure, conflicts).

In order to accomplish these main goals, the therapist undertakes the following therapeutic interventions:

1. Meet the patient, start binge/purge charts, and weigh the patient.
2. Meet the rest of the family in a sincere and warm manner.
3. Take a history that elicits from each family member how he/she has been impacted by the eating disorder.
4. Separate the illness from the patient.
5. Orchestrate an intense scene to convey the seriousness of the illness and the difficulty in recovery.
6. Prepare the parents and the adolescent for the meal the following week and end the session.

Clinical Background

Jenny is a 17-year-old Caucasian female presenting with a diagnosis of BN. Her height is 63 inches, and her weight is 111.5 pounds with a body mass index (BMI) of 19.8. She is currently residing with her parents and younger brother (Peter). She also has an older sister (Mandy) who lives away at college. Jenny presented to the clinic with bulimic symptoms that began 12 months ago, and she reports binge eating 10 times in the past 4 weeks and purging every other day over the same time period. Jenny does not report using laxatives, diuretics, or diet pills, but she engaged in compensatory exercise approximately once a week in the last month. This exercise includes running and other aerobic workouts. Jenny has missed one menstrual cycle in the last 3 months and is not taking oral contraceptives. She denied any functional impairment due to her eating disorder.

Meet the Patient, Start Binge/Purge Charts, and Weigh the Patient

Prior to beginning the session, the therapist walked Jenny to her office, weighed her (she is wearing light indoor clothing), and asked about her binge and purging frequency during the prior week. Jenny's answer was carefully noted on the therapist's *binge/purge charts* (see previous chapter for detail). During this process, the therapist briefly discussed with Jenny her feelings about beginning therapy.

Meet the Rest of the Family in a Sincere and Warm Manner

Although this family has three other members living at home, only Mother accompanied her daughter to this session. Father was away on business and Mother was reluctant to have Jenny's younger sibling join them for this session. She held to her view, despite the therapist's initial efforts to convince both parents that it would be essential for all family members living at home to attend this meeting. The therapist nevertheless proceeded with the first session and upon greeting the mother, expressed her worry that the husband could not join her today. The therapist then said how she was looking forward to her (Mother) relaying the essence of this meeting to Dad and meeting him and their son the following week. Despite the absence of both the father and the son, the therapist made sure that she explored their probable viewpoints of the adolescent's illness in this session. Also, she made sure to impress upon Mother and daughter how important it will be to have everyone attend Session 2.

Take a History That Elicits from Each Family Member How He/She Has Been Impacted by the Eating Disorder

THERAPIST: Jenny, I know a little bit about you from what our team wrote in the assessment process that you went through, but I would like to know more about you and how your life has changed since you've had this eating disorder—and, likewise, how your [family] life has changed because that's the reason we feel it's really important to involve parents and your sister and your brother. I would be glad if they can join us in the treatment because the eating disorder not only affects Jenny, it affects all of you.

MOTHER: Can I interrupt?

THERAPIST: Sure.

MOTHER: Her brother knows nothing about this. He has no idea why we're going to therapy, or anything like that, and I don't know that I want him to know.

THERAPIST: Okay.

MOTHER: You know, her sister, that's a different story. I don't think I mind if Peter knows that Jenny has trouble with food, with her relationship to food and all that kind of stuff, because he sees that she eats a ton of fruit. But I don't see the benefit of him knowing any more detail. And it's the same with my extended family. I just don't see why that matters. I wouldn't want [Peter] to know.

THERAPIST: Jenny, what's your perspective on what your mom said?

JENNY: Um.

THERAPIST: You know your brother really well, obviously.

JENNY: Yes, I think it might be uncomfortable.

THERAPIST: For you to have him here?

JENNY: Yes, well, I don't know if he would handle it well or if he wouldn't—I don't think he'd really voice much of an opinion.

THERAPIST: Uh-huh.

JENNY: So I think it might be better . . .

THERAPIST: Well, why don't we do this: Why don't we suspend a decision on that until the end of the session today? I obviously want to respect your need to do what's best for your family and what makes you feel the most comfortable. Let me give you a sense of what the treatment looks like, and we can talk a little bit more about that in the end.

MOTHER: All right.

JENNY: Uh-huh.

THERAPIST: That's good. Well, I guess I should back up and say that I specialize in eating disorders. In particular, for the past few years I have worked pretty much exclusively with adolescents who have eating disorders. So I really hope that I'll be able to help you as you help your daughter get better from this illness. But really what I'm curious about knowing is, Jenny, how having bulimia has affected your life. Tell me a little bit more about when it started, and what came next.

JENNY: Uh-huh.

THERAPIST: (*turning to the mother*) Feel free to jump in too. This doesn't have to be a "you go, then you go."

MOTHER: Okay.

JENNY: Yeah, I guess it's hard to say how it affected my life because it just happened, and there's just not that much, it just like happened in 1 day, so there's not much difference between that day and the next.

THERAPIST: I see. What occurred first? Maybe tell me about when you really knew that there was something going on, something other than just being concerned about eating.

JENNY: Well, I sort of had a problem in, what, seventh grade?

THERAPIST: Uh-huh.

MOTHER: You weren't eating at all basically.

JENNY: Yeah.

MOTHER: And she got really skinny. What stands out in my mind is, we went to South Carolina, to the beach, and she was just a stick, and she was also very uncommunicative and just not herself.

THERAPIST: Okay.

MOTHER: I don't know if we were aware of your problem then or if it was right after you got back. It was in that time period.

JENNY: Uh-huh.

MOTHER: She was just a different person, and then after she started eating again we went and saw the doctor.

JENNY: Yeah.

MOTHER: And she took to heart what the doctor had to say and started eating again, and she just bounced right back—I mean, the personality change was dramatic.

THERAPIST: Okay. When she was at a very low body weight, it was different from when she was obviously healthy?

MOTHER: Yeah.

JENNY: Yeah.

MOTHER: She seemed to respond well to what the doctor had to say, and she started drinking protein shakes.

JENNY: Yeah, I made myself protein smoothies and stuff. Then I went into eighth grade and when I was a freshman and sophomore—I guess around sophomore year—I've always been really concerned. I don't know exactly when it started—this is really scary—because I know a lot of girls who have thrown up what they eat just sometimes, just to try it, for whatever reason. I started in the summer after sophomore year, I think, and then this year it's just gotten progressively worse and noticeably since maybe February, it was just getting really bad. I'm not going to summer camp 'cause I can't control it.

THERAPIST: Okay.

JENNY: So, I don't really know how it's affected my life. When it got really bad is also when summer started. Every other year I've been going to this camp in the summer because there's not much to do. So I think that changed my life. I'm not going to get to do that, and maybe it has an effect on my life.

THERAPIST: I see, so having a lot of time on your hands actually caused the illness to get worse?

JENNY: That's what I think.

MOTHER: Then what happened is that she'd get depressed about the fact that she has this "thing," and she would do even less. So it's sort of a vicious circle.

THERAPIST: Yes, very much so. I think that that's what a lot of patients who feel depressed would say. Do you see that? What do you do when your parents get concerned? Or if your mom gets worried about you and your health, what are some things that you really have noticed that you do?

Note that the therapist includes the father in the discussions about how the eating disorder impacted the parents. Although Dad may, of course, have a different viewpoint than Mother, the therapist nevertheless makes sure that he is "present" in the session in some way. Mother's response is to make an effort to let the therapist know about joint thoughts or decisions with her husband regarding Jenny's illness.

JENNY: There's nothing, It's not about her being overconcerned. I came to my mom because I started getting scared and . . .

THERAPIST: About the bingeing and the purging?

JENNY: Yeah.

MOTHER: Yeah. Yes, her sister mentioned it to my husband and me, it must have been last summer . . .

THERAPIST: (to Jenny) Because she had heard you?

MOTHER: Yeah.

JENNY: Yeah.

MOTHER: I guess we didn't take it seriously, so when I mentioned it to Mandy this summer, she's like "Mom, I told you guys." It's been hard for us to monitor Jenny. I knew that the food thing was getting out of hand, with the summer . . .

THERAPIST: Yeah.

MOTHER: Or late this spring into summer, but I didn't know why, until she came to me. And I guess I should do more. What I feel like I should do is just to be more noticing of anything else she's up to and just be around for her more. I think both my husband and I have been trying to do that, although the last couple weeks she's stayed at a girlfriend's.

THERAPIST: Okay, well I think one of the really positive indicators is that Jenny, you were able to feel confident and comfortable, for lack of a better word, in coming to your mom, and I think that also shows a lot of bravery on your part and also motivation to get better from this. It's a really positive indicator, and I'm very glad that you're feeling that because I, of course, agree.

MOTHER: And that's when we went to the doctor, and she talked about medication and depression and all that, and, like you said, Jenny was able to confront this, and she wants to help find a cure. So I just can't think that Jenny is, you know, depressed.

THERAPIST: Okay.

MOTHER: She might have a different feeling, you know, inside her, but I think that those outward signs are really good. She's a fighter and she wants to get this.

Although Mother's praise for her daughter's fighting spirit is welcome, the astute therapist will make sure to what extent the bulimia is indeed experienced as ego dystonic by the adolescent. If the patient expressed the wish to "get this," it is important to move forward with great caution when the parents are assigned the task of helping their daughter fight the illness and not assume that the adolescent can do this by herself. The parent also makes the important point that her daughter might be depressed. The therapist's task is to not let the issue of a potential comorbidity derail the attention to the eating disorder, but, at the same time, also not to overlook an obvious issue that might be causing the patient considerable distress, and if not addressed, will derail the treatment down the line. If there is indeed a comorbid depression, the therapist will try to learn more about it by making a referral to the child and adolescent psychiatrist on the team.

THERAPIST: Well, I think that's really great. Sometimes eating disorders are complicated, very complicated, illnesses and certain other conditions coexist with them, such as depression and anxiety. So if ever that's something of concern that all of us notice and that we could deal with that through the clinic, we will want to be able to make sure . . .

MOTHER: Anxiety (*nervous laughter*).

THERAPIST: Right, right, but we're really targeting the bulimia, and the other things often improve. I've seen that in patients that I've worked with; they might have depression or anxiety, but actually when you work on getting them better from the eating disorder, the other things improve as well. So let's just take it one therapy session at a time. It's really helpful for me to know where both of you are coming from and to have more of a background in terms of how the eating disorder developed.

MOTHER: My husband also knows about it, and he's expressed to me that he's happy with her for doing this because he feels like he doesn't know what he should be doing too, so he's kind of helpless.

Separate the Illness from the Patient

Here the therapist attempts to emphasize that the adolescent and the eating disorder are two separate entities (even when the adolescent claims that she IS the eating disorder, and vice versa). The therapist's goal is twofold: in so doing, she/he is alleviating the guilt the parents may feel in having caused the illness; bulimia is no different from any other illness, medical or psychiatric. The second reason for separating the illness from the adolescent is to enable everyone (parents and patient) to be able to aim their efforts *at* the illness, as opposed to at the adolescent, when the therapist enlists everyone's energy in fighting the symptomatic behavior. There are several ways to separate the illness from the adolescent: The therapist can allude to bulimia as being no different from a malignant tumor. It is something that developed, outside the adolescent's control, and if left untreated, can and will cause incredible harm. Each therapist, though, should find the best metaphor that sits comfortably with him/her as therapist and one that will be understood and appreciated by the family.

THERAPIST: Okay. Working with a lot of families, I've seen parents come with different emotions or feelings about their daughter or their son who gets diagnosed with an eating disorder. I think one of the common things that parents say is, "What did I do to cause this?" They'll feel a lot of guilt. You said something earlier about "We didn't take it seriously, when Mandy. . . . "

MOTHER: Uh-huh.

THERAPIST: Mandy, your other daughter, had come and told you that she was concerned about her sister. I think the most important point for everyone in this room to know is that *no one caused this eating disorder.* We don't know how eating disorders develop. Hopefully in 5 years' time or 10 years' time we'll be able to more definitively figure out why this happens to girls like your daughter. It's probably very complicated, it's probably multideterminant, and we don't have a solution at the moment. And the causes are probably very unique for each person. So what may cause an eating disorder in your daughter may not be the cause of the eating disorder in the next patient that I see in the clinic. What we really know is that parents are not responsible for causing this illness. Just from the little information I have on you, I've already determined that you're very caring parents, and that you want to make sure that Jenny gets better from this, and that you want to be able to know how to help her. Instead of viewing parents as somehow causing this illness, we view you as the best resource, because we feel that no one else is an expert on Jenny the way you and your husband are. That's why we really want to utilize you as a resource and involve you in every step of the way in Jenny's treatment, and that's why I'm so glad you came in tonight and got her in for treatment, and that Jenny was brave enough to tell you what was going on.

So these are all, as I said earlier, indications of her getting better. The other point is that it's really important to tackle eating disorders early on because we know that the longer you let them go without treating them, the harder they are to treat. So I think all the more reason that I'm glad I work in a child and adolescent clinic, and that I see a lot of adolescents who are at the very early stage of the illness. I think it's easier to treat any type of illness if it's early on in its expression. I keep using the word *illness* for *bulimia*, and I don't know if perhaps that seems a little strange or foreign to people. The reason I do that is because I know that it's not your daughter who's bingeing on food or getting rid of it afterward; she would never do that. She strikes me as being someone you can count on, rely on; she's trustworthy, not secretive; she doesn't hide things. Are these statements all true about your daughter or not?

MOTHER: Uh-huh.

THERAPIST: And so I know that she knows that it's unhealthy to be doing these types of behaviors. I think you said something earlier about it being foreign to you, that it was out of control. I forget, which term did you use?

JENNY: Oh, okay, out of control.

THERAPIST: And so it's not Jenny who's in control of the symptoms, it's really this illness that gets her to do these things that she knows are unhealthy, this bingeing and purging that are really detrimental to her health. That's why I refer to it as *the illness* or *bulimia* because this illness came upon her and now it's up to all of us to deal with it and to figure out how to take it away from her.

MOTHER: Right.

THERAPIST: I think it's also helpful to view it as something separate from your daughter, something that is its own illness. It's just like, if she were to have cancer, a tumor, it would affect how she felt. That tumor is called bulimia nervosa.

MOTHER: Uh-huh.

THERAPIST: So, with you and your husband's continued and really energetic efforts, you can work to get Jenny back without her eating disorder. I don't know if you had questions about that point specifically?—about making the distinction between how much of Jenny is doing this and how much of this is bulimia that's doing this. From my perspective and my experience working with families, it's 100% the illness that gets her to act in this way, this sort of secretive or sneaky bingeing or purging.

The therapist wants to make sure that the parents really *get* the distinction between their daughter and the illness. In addition to the goals for this distinction mentioned earlier, by making it clear that these symptoms are outside the adolescent's control, the therapist also helps the parents view their daughter's struggle without criticism. Although she (the adolescent) can aid in her own recovery, she is not to blame for bingeing and purging.

MOTHER: Uh-huh.

THERAPIST: (*turning to Jenny*) You strike me as a very logical individual, and you know that these are not healthy behaviors you're engaging in.

MOTHER: It's true, and I know that, you know, she just expressed that she can't control it. And you know, maybe that's one of the scariest parts. But, yeah, when you say it is an illness, it's hard for me to grasp that, because it doesn't have the physical component that cancer does.

THERAPIST: That you can identify the tumor?

MOTHER: Yeah.

THERAPIST: I think, probably in 5 years' time, 10 years' time, we will be able to know more biologically about why it is that your daughter has an eating disorder and figuring out what sort of complex brain mechanism is involved that makes a person have an eating disorder. It's a specialty, so we're treating this illness just the way we would treat cancer.

MOTHER: I have a question. When did, when did these eating disorders come on the scene?

THERAPIST: I think that's a great question. We're really in our infancy in terms of researching them and understanding them and treating them. It was Gerald Russell who originally termed the concept of bulimia nervosa in 1979, so it's been pretty recent that this has actually been looked at. We have historical records of the behaviors themselves occurring in the Middle Ages and what not, but no one had really diagnosed it as bulimia nervosa, per se, or as a medical problem, an illness—just like major depression. So bulimia has been around officially since 1979, in diagnosis textbooks and literature. Since then, a lot of research has gone into looking at how to best treat bulimia nervosa. Most of the research has focused on adults, and that's why it's very fortunate that we have this opportunity to study how best to treat adolescents with bulimia. Adolescents are very different from adults, so we might have to treat them with a different type of treatment than we use with adults.

MOTHER: Uh-huh.

THERAPIST: It's a good question. I think it also speaks to the fact that we're continuing to figure out what it is that causes these illnesses and how we can best treat them. And as I said before, we know that involving parents in the treatment process with anorexia is incredibly beneficial. So that's why we have every reason to think that including both of you in the treatment actively will help Jenny. I don't know how much homework or research you've done, or how many doctors' visits and if they spelled out all the ways in which bulimia nervosa really is harmful. You know, I alluded to it earlier, of you being a very logical individual and knowing that these are harmful behaviors you're engaging in.

MOTHER: We went to the doctor and she talked to us. (*turning to Jenny*) I don't know if you've done any research on the Internet, I really haven't.

JENNY: No, well, just the stuff from the doctor.

Orchestrate an Intense Scene

In the following passages the therapist will make every effort to let the Jenny and her mother register the full extent to which the eating disorder has already impacted Jenny's physical as well as psychological health. Likewise, she will also alert them to the ways in which this illness can further cause Jenny to suffer in these domains. In doing so, the therapist is attempting to raise the mother's concerns about the severity of the illness so that she is enabled to take more concrete action in helping her daughter fight the illness. For all cases it is vitally important for the therapist to make a careful assessment of the parents' (when both are present) current level of anxiety around these issues and to only raise their concerns to a level that will enable them to take the next step in helping their daughter. Making parents too anxious about the consequences of the illness could contribute to their feeling guilt and/or immobilize them in their efforts.

THERAPIST: I'm most likely going to be reiterating a lot of what the doctor probably told you. I'm a big believer in the more times you hear something, the more it will really sink in—the gravity of this problem. It affects many different mechanisms; it affects a person physically. Every time Jenny purges, the stomach acids from the vomit that comes out not only can erode the esophagus, so you actually get esophageal tears.

And I've had individuals report there's blood in their vomit, and this is something that we take very seriously. They needed to go to the emergency room right away, because the blood could be indicating an actual tear in the esophagus. And then the other thing that the stomach acids erode every time you vomit in addition to the esophagus, is the enamel on your teeth. And that can be irreversible, causing a lot of dental problems and periodontal disease later on, but right away you can have problems with cavities because you lack enamel on your teeth, because that's been eroded away.

Also, frequent vomiting can really wreak havoc on your electrolyte system, particularly your potassium. Electrolytes are really important because, simply put, they tell the heart to beat. So you can see a lot of cardiac problems with bulimia. A person can complain that she is feeling faint and dizzy because she doesn't have enough potassium circulating in the system; and this is worsened by purging. Every time that you purge, you disrupt your body's natural electrolyte levels. That's very, very serious, and I think the very scary thing is that we don't know how many times someone has to vomit or purge to get an esophageal tear or a wearing away of the esophagus, or how many times they have to vomit before their enamel wears off their teeth. What we do know is that every time you do this, you're putting your body in jeopardy of these things happening. I talked about cardiac problems as the result of the electrolyte disturbances. You can see lower heart beat or irregular heart beats—substantial cardiac problems—associated with bingeing and purging. The eating behaviors are inherently very shameful and secretive and can affect you psychologically, which is why I'm so very glad you have a good relationship with your mom and dad, that you felt comfortable telling them about this problem. I know that these are not behaviors that you want to have or that you're proud of. I know that you know that there's something wrong with engaging in these behaviors, that they can also lead to a really severe preoccupation with your body shape and weight with preoccupied thoughts about, "When am I going to be able to binge next?", "When am I going to get rid of all the calories?"—your constant mind-set is on food or eating or shape. You're the one who's directly affected by this problem. These things I just mentioned—the preoccupations—are psychological. Are they true?

MOTHER: Well, yeah.

JENNY: Yeah.

THERAPIST: And your mom can talk about it as well.

JENNY: Yeah, well, I don't know. It's hard to tell what came first. I think it's hard to identify in myself because I don't notice the thoughts. I'm just normal to myself because it seems like I worry about things, but it's not out of the ordinary or it doesn't seem like I could have eaten another way. So, I don't know.

THERAPIST: Uh-huh. (*turning to the mother*) What is it like for you to hear Jenny talk about her illness? Is this something you heard before from the pediatrician?

MOTHER: The things that you were talking about?

THERAPIST: Yeah, the negative ways in which the eating disorder can really . . .

MOTHER: Yeah.

THERAPIST: They're very serious.

MOTHER: Yeah.

THERAPIST: Life threatening.

MOTHER: I would think that it would kind of scare Jenny . . .

THERAPIST: (*to Jenny*) Does it feel scary to hear that these are the medical and psychological risks associated with bingeing and purging?

JENNY: I heard about the risks from health class in school and the other doctor. I guess it's weird to be able to identify it in myself, and maybe I don't take it seriously enough, but I do understand.

THERAPIST: Uh-huh. Well, I think in some ways, there's almost a quality of invincibility in a thought, "Oh, maybe that'll happen to someone else, but that won't happen to me." A lot of patients have made that kind of statement to me. And I think that's really the scary thing about bulimia. I work with patients who haven't had the symptoms for a very long time—maybe only 5 or 6 months, and they have had blood in their vomit. I worked with one individual who collapsed on the basketball court. She was a great basketball player, but she had been bingeing and purging, which led to incredibly low potassium and she became dizzy and fainted.

MOTHER: Which you do sometimes . . .

JENNY: I don't . . . well, I guess . . . it's hard to, again, try to respond.

THERAPIST: Right.

JENNY: Plus, the doctor said that a lot of damage would be longer term.

MOTHER: Right.

JENNY: Yeah, right.

THERAPIST: I would agree with the doctor. I think that there are certain longer term effects. We've done studies and found that there could be menstrual irregularities. I don't know if there's any research looking into fertility and how that's affected by bulimia. You know, there's a lot of research with anorexia. I think the very positive point about both anorexia and bulimia is that if you attack them early enough and really aggressively treat them so that you get better, improve, and are in the recovery phase, then you don't have to worry about them as much. They're not going to be creeping up on you later in life. If you can stop the bingeing and the purging, then you're not putting your body at risk. I often say to patients that it's like they're playing Russian roulette with their body in essence. Every time you purge, there's a possibility of a negative consequence.

MOTHER: But I think that when she said long term, she thought this whole corrosive effect and you're saying . . .

THERAPIST: Everybody's esophagus and teeth are different, and there's not really one formula that says that someone has to have these symptoms for 1 year or 5 years for there to be any damage.

MOTHER: Uh-huh.

THERAPIST: Some people experience an incredible amount of damage in 6 months from bingeing and purging. It seems very innocuous or very seductive to say, "I think this will be the last time that I do this, I won't do this ever again." Like you said earlier, when we started talking: You said that it's a vicious cycle and it ends up controlling you as opposed to you feeling like you're in control of it. Well, I realize I have unloaded all of this on you, and part of the reason for doing this is that we know what we're up against, and you know how powerful this illness can be and how serious it is at that same time. And so it's very scary, I realize, to hear those things, for Jenny and for you as her parents. But the thing we really have going for us is that you and your husband care about her so very much and are experts on your own family and would like to be able to be more involved in helping her get better from this. Your husband had said to me, just even out in the hall [the therapist met the father at the time of the assessment], "I really believe in this treatment and I want to be able to do whatever I can do to help make sure she's okay."

MOTHER: Uh-huh.

The therapist reviewed the consequences of the eating disorder very carefully and charged the parents (even though the father wasn't present), in collaboration with their offspring, with the task of working together to make sure that the illness is defeated. Throughout the session, the therapist remained respectful of the adolescent's concerns about her autonomy, but made sure to get the point across that there is perhaps no other way forward than the one suggested by the therapist. In the following passages, the therapist will become somewhat more specific in terms of what has to happen around mealtimes to bring about symptomatic relief.

Charge the Parents and the Adolescent with the Task of Regular Eating without Bingeing and Purging

THERAPIST: So, that's really where you as parents come in and what your important role is in this treatment. As I mentioned to you, we've learned that parents are really incredibly successful in getting their children back to healthy weight in anorexia and in much the same way we believe that parents can be the most effective at helping arrest the bingeing and purging in bulimia. That's really the task of this treatment, and I realize it's not an easy thing for you to do. I know it probably feels a bit like "This is not something I ought to be doing for my daughter, who is this young woman and should be in control of when she eats and how much she eats and when she goes to the bathroom."

MOTHER: Uh-huh.

THERAPIST: You and your husband are up against a really tough illness, so you need to be stronger than the illness and have a treatment that is 10 times stronger than the illness. Essentially I'm putting the success if this treatment in both of your laps, you and your husband's: Your role is to really help Jenny, *with* Jenny's help, get better from this. Do you have a question?

MOTHER: Well, when you said, "What kind of changes in Jenny," and then you're talking about that we take a much more active role in everyday function?

THERAPIST: Right.

MOTHER: It sounds like . . .

THERAPIST: If I could just add one thing so that Jenny doesn't hyperventilate, because I know every adolescent I see will hear what I'm saying and think, "They're siccing my parents on me! They're going to be in control of every single aspect of my life!" (*turning to the mother*) Not at all; you and your husband are only in control of the eating aspect.

So you're there to help her with anything regarding what she's eating or if she's maybe getting rid of it by going to the bathroom.

MOTHER: Be helpful, right. What I was going to comment on is that I felt like this year Jenny was not paying attention in her schoolwork like she has in the past. We're both kind of hands-off parents. We have one older kid who is real easy, a really good kid, and I pretty much let her do whatever she wants, because she knows what she's doing. But this past year Jenny has been really preoccupied with running, working out, and that whole thing, and not focused on her schoolwork. So I don't know how much that has to do with the illness, but when you're saying we'll be in charge of Jenny's eating, I also feel like there's that other component that what she does in her free time is kind of excessive. She really has to work out or she gets pissed.

THERAPIST: Well, let me mention, that's also part of it. This treatment is different from the treatment for anorexia, where the immediate goal is to restore weight to a healthy level. Someone with bulimia has weight that is within a normal range, so what we're trying to do is help her make healthy decisions regarding her eating, make sure that her eating is regular, and make sure that she doesn't purge afterward. One form of purging actually can be overexercising. I work with another family where the adolescent does not vomit but engages in excessive exercise, so her parents help to monitor that and make sure that it's not over and above what it would be healthy for someone Jenny's age. We're not at all saying, "I forbid you, Jenny, from exercising." It's just you want to be able to shift the thinking so that you're exercising because it's healthy, you don't overdo it, and you enjoy it—as opposed to exercising because "I want to burn x number of calories" or to have your mind be preoccupied with "How many calories am I burning" or "I have to do it for 45 minutes or an hour, not just half an hour." There's sort of a compulsive quality to it.

(to the mother) I think that in addition to helping Jenny at mealtime, you can also make sure that she's not tempted to listen to what the bulimia would tell her to do—which is, "Go to the bathroom, get rid of that, you ate too much," or "Go run to get rid of it." You and your husband can fulfill an incredibly pivotal role in helping her not do this. And the wonderful thing is that, Jenny, you don't want to be doing this and you want help with this. And while everyone differs and some people may be able to do this on their own, I also know that who better than your parents knows you so well? No one else is as invested in your well-being and love you as much as your parents do. And so just as if Jenny has cancer and you know you have to take care of her—help her through chemotherapy or radiation, or make sure that she takes her medicine everyday—these are just things you do as a parent. Likewise with bulimia, the problem is different, but it's no less serious. She's bingeing and purging, and she's putting her body at excess risk for all of these things we've talked about. And so you and your husband can lovingly help her with this particular area, while I function as your consultant, helping you do this. But I think, for the most part, you already know what you need to do as her parents.

In these preceding passages the therapist made sure to spell out the role of the parents in helping their daughter with her eating disorder. She also made sure to let both mother and daughter know that the role is both temporary and limited to eating and purging behaviors, all the while being respectful of Jenny's concerns about this proposed parental task. In fact, the therapist made sure to let the adolescent know she is also part of her own recovery (with her parents' help), whereas the role of the therapist is that of a consultant to the family. In the following passages the therapist continues along this track and works hard to make sure that she compliments the mother on her and her husband's knowledge not only of their child, but what needs to happen in order for her to recover from the eating disorder (i.e., empowering the parents).

THERAPIST: That's what I'm here to do, to help you think through what you think you ought to do. Unfortunately, what an eating disorder does to parents, in particular, and to the adolescents who are affected by it, is it trips them up and it makes them think "I can't help my child/ myself get better from this." I may be the professional in this room, but ultimately you and your husband will be the ones who will help her figure this out. You know her the best of anyone, and you don't need to be told what is a healthy amount of food for someone of Jenny's age to be eating. And you don't need to be told that it's unhealthy for her to be getting rid of it in the bathroom. And you know when she's overexercising, you know all these things. I think part of my job is just to remind you that you know all this and to help you along the way by supporting you to make sure that you continue to fight the good fight so that your intervention is 10 times stronger than this tumor called bulimia nervosa. I've talked a lot today. The first session I end up talking the most, but as we go along, you guys will be talking more.

MOTHER: Yeah, it's daunting. What I anticipate is arguments, you know, because it's not something easy.

THERAPIST: You're right on that, and Jenny, I value so much your perspective on this because you're the one who is affected by this. Everyone else is affected by this of course, but no one else is affected in the way that you are affected by it. And your role is to let your parents know how they can help you, to figure out a way that's comfortable for you, so it doesn't feel like it's invasive. But I absolutely understand that you're a teenager, so part of your teenage DNA is to be rebellious against your parents and not want them to help you and do the opposite of what they say. I don't want to take that away (*then jokingly to the mother*) . . . maybe your mom and dad would like me to take that away from you.

MOTHER: No . . . (*laughing*).

THERAPIST: I don't want to take that away from you. All I want your parents to do is really take away the bulimia from you. I work with a lot of families and they've been able to take away the bulimia, through the help of their adolescent. You have a really important part of educating your parents about what works. So let them know if there is a way for them to help you that's more comfortable for you, as opposed to taking all the doors off the hinges of every bathroom in your house. You know, there's ways to do it that will obviously make you feel uncomfortable, and ways in which they can do it that will make you feel like you're supported and that they're on your side, and really what all of you're up against is the bulimia. (*turning to the mother*) You're up against the bulimia, you're not up against Jenny. You're actually helping Jenny by helping her make these decisions. Right now, unfortunately, when it comes to eating, it's the bulimia that dictates. And when you said you anticipate some potential arguments, then know that you're battling the bulimia, you're having an argument with bulimia, and that's why I think it's really helpful that you separate the two: your daughter and the bulimia.

MOTHER: When you said, as far as you know, Jenny wants to cure this—I think one of the hardest things is to dictate her workout schedule.

THERAPIST: Okay.

MOTHER: I think that she is pretty invested in doing these things, and she'll be psychologically struggling.

THERAPIST: We can do whatever is most comfortable for you. It can be a step-by-step process in which you work on the purging specifically and then work on the exercising a little bit. But really tackle one problem at a time. There's going to be, of course, bumps along the way; bulimia is a very selfish illness, and it's only happy when it gets its way. Unfortunately, sometimes the illness robs someone with an eating disorder of her ability to see that it is a problem and it is serious. And I'm very happy that your daughter has insight into how dangerous this is and how these are very unpleasant behaviors. I feel incredibly confident that we all will be able to help her. In regard to having your son come in, I wanted to get back to that issue. Your sister, Jenny, and your brother serve very different roles than your parents. While your parents are going to be helping you get better, so that you don't binge or that you don't purge or overexercise . . .

JENNY: Uh-huh.

Wanting to remind the family (in this case, the mother and Jenny) that everyone has a role to play in Jenny's recovery, the therapist makes sure to bring everyone who lives at home into the picture here and spells out everyone's role in moving forward. This is especially important because the father and brother did not show up for Session 1. Although the therapist has already spelled out to the mother what her and her husband's role will be, she also takes some time to help the mother understand that her son also has an important role in Jenny's treatment. If he is to be his sister's ally, then it would be helpful to get to know him a little and makes sure he understands how he can be helpful. This is an issue that the therapist will revisit before the session is over to impress upon the mother and Jenny that she expects to see all four of them present for Session 2. Therapists should always set this expectation but be respectful if they (parents) really don't want to bring other siblings along.

THERAPIST: Your brother and your sister—even if she's away at college, there's still a phone and there's still e-mail—are there to support you. This is going be tough, and there are going to be times when you're going to be mad at your mom and dad because they're saying that you can't go to the bathroom after you eat. It will be important for you to be able to go to your brother or say to your sister on the phone, "I can't stand Mom and Dad! Why are they doing this to me! It feels like they're controlling my life!" Their role is *not* to be the one saying,

"Jenny, I saw you go to the bathroom" or "Jenny, I saw that you ate too much fruit." In that way it may be helpful, but, again, I'll leave it to your discretion whether or not your son comes in. I really want to be respectful of the fact that it's not something that you want.

MOTHER: Well, it's just interesting to think about my son in a supporting role because, I mean, he's the youngest, and he's got his own issues. He could actually be a very supportive person, but we just don't know that side of him. So I don't know, I think that's maybe something we'll have to talk about.

THERAPIST: It can definitely be an open invitation too. So if you feel like, early on, you don't necessarily want him, he can also come later when the eating disorder it a little more under control. I just want to make sure, Jenny, that you have somewhere you can feel supported. So if that support isn't found in your brother, that's okay?

JENNY: Uh-huh.

THERAPIST: It could be found in good girlfriends or someone you feel comfortable talking to. It doesn't even have to be that you call them up or sit down with them to talk, and say, "I'm really worried because I think I'm going to binge or I'm going to purge." Sometimes it's just helpful to have someone other than your parents you can vent to about having a bad day.

JENNY: Right.

THERAPIST: Can we talk about it?

JENNY: When I binge and then go to sleep, I don't want to gain weight.

THERAPIST: This is the hardest part for you, and I know that the fear is that you're going to gain so much weight on this program. I think the most important thing is that that's not what anyone's goal is in here. What we want is to see you maintain a healthy weight, and we want to see that your eating is under control and that you're not having this urge to go to the toilet afterward. From my own experiences of the families I've worked with, none of the girls has gained much weight at all. In fact, some of them stay the same weight, some of them gain maybe something, not much, like 5 pounds at most. Believe me, I would have to rethink being a therapist if treatment were causing people to gain a lot of weight. We definitely don't want that. What we really want to do is figure out a way that you can sit down and have a normal amount of fruit that doesn't lead to bingeing. That's where your mom and your dad are going to be really helpful, because they love you so much they're not going to let it turn into a binge.

In the preceding passage the therapist makes an effort to reassure the adolescent that the main goal of this treatment is to help her be healthy again and on track with adolescent development. This is an issue that may very well have to be revisited several times, because it is highly unlikely and unrealistic to expect the adolescent's fears around weight and shape issues to dissipate so soon in treatment. The therapist shows great respect and sympathy for the adolescent here, which most probably will pay dividends as treatment proceeds and the relationship between the adolescent and therapist is put to the test.

MOTHER: Well, actually, she doesn't, she doesn't purge fruit.
THERAPIST: Oh.
MOTHER: That's her safe food.
JENNY: I don't even know. But I don't want to. If you like catch me at the end or something, because I don't want to purge because that'll make me more anxious.
THERAPIST: Yeah, well I think part of this is it's the illness that's so afraid, because it gets you to purge. I know it may sound crazy, but maybe by the end of this you'll say, "Okay, now I know what she was talking about when she kept calling it the illness or bulimia or whatever." We can name it something else, if you want to. We don't have to call it *bulimia* or *illness*, but this thing, this bulimia, it gets you to be so terrified of weight—"Oh, my gosh, I can't keep this down, this is way too much food, I'm going to gain an incredible amount of weight"—and that's not the case. Everyone has periods of time in which they overeat, but they don't necessarily feel the urge to get rid of it. So what really we're wanting to do is make sure that you don't feel like you're overeating. First of all, we want you to be able to eat a normal amount of food or a regular amount of food, and that's where your mom and dad don't need to have me or a nutritionist tell them exactly what it is you should be eating. I know this because Mandy, your sister, looked very healthy, and your brother looked healthy [the therapist met every family member at the assessment session]. I know that they already know what would be a good amount of food for you to have on your plate when you have dinner or what's a healthy snack, what's a healthy lunch, breakfast.

  Believe me, no one in this room wants you to feel miserable, so we have to figure out a way in which you can help us help you. You need to tell us what helps and what doesn't help because you're a collaborator in this—not that I'm going to be talking just to your mom and dad and excluding you from the conversation, not at all. You have a very important role in saying how the week went, what you'd like for your parents to do to help you, what you feel you need some more guidance with, what times are really hard for you when you're especially afraid that you might binge or purge, and are there specific foods that your mom and dad can help you eat again? Maybe not having them around for a bit of time might be easier. We could make a guess about what might be helpful, but the best thing would be if you could tell us when it's hard and what foods are hard so that we can figure out how to make it not so hard for you to eat a normal amount of them, and for you to walk away from the table and not even have an idea that you need to get rid of what you've just eaten.

JENNY: I guess I get afraid that I might binge, so I just don't eat for like a long time. Then it's easier to . . . like when I'm really hungry and there's sometimes I just don't eat for a long period of time and it starts with food and . . .

THERAPIST: Okay, I see.

JENNY: And then fruit fills you, but it doesn't decrease your appetite really, and then I don't know.

THERAPIST: Okay, I guess I understand now.

JENNY: So I guess the fruit triggers the bingeing.

THERAPIST: So it sounds like already you've, just in Session 1 already figured out what triggers the bingeing. This is something families sometimes don't discover until later on. These are all things that are incredibly helpful for all of us to know. The best thing is for you to feel like you can talk about this stuff and that it's not going to backfire and you're going to lose control. You want bulimia to lose control, the control it has over you, and I want you to feel more control over eating. I know right now it's so scary to have to sit in the kitchen, fearful of overeating, or thinking "I'm going to eat too much of this" or "I have to get rid of this, I've eaten too much." No one needs to have to wrestle with that on her own.

JENNY: Okay.

THERAPIST: Okay. Well, I know I've laid a lot on you, and believe me, as we go along with this treatment, we'll be able to spell out more clearly what each individual role is. Practically speaking, it's you and your husband who are going to make sure that Jenny's eating becomes normal again, so she doesn't have to binge and she doesn't have to purge.

What would be really helpful for us is, the next time that we meet, for as many people that can be here, to come. It's really up to you if you feel like you want your son to come. If your husband can come, that would be great.

MOTHER: We could do that.

Prepare the Family for the Next Session's Meal and Closing the Session

It is crucially important that all family members living at home with the patient be present for the following treatment sessions. The therapist makes it quite clear then in these final minutes of the session to stress that she's expecting the presence of everyone next time round. Neither the mother nor Jenny voiced any opposition.

THERAPIST: Let me tell you just a little bit about the second time that we meet. We usually like to have families bring in what would be a typical dinner, if we're meeting in the early evening. One of the reasons we do it this way is that I can't come into your house and see how a dinner goes.

MOTHER: So you want us to bring *food*?

THERAPIST: I want you and your husband to bring in a meal that would set your daughter on the path to recovery, so that the two of you can establish healthy eating patterns. There's one extra expectation—I want you to bring in something that's difficult for Jenny to eat on her own, something that might be a forbidden food item and that may typically lead to a binge if she were to eat any of it. For some young women that may be a sweet dessert, for instance. So, bring in something that you and Jenny's dad could help her eat in the session. It doesn't have to be a large amount, but something that would be hard to eat, so that you are able to have the experience of helping her feel comfortable eating things that are hard to eat. Does that make sense? You had said the 16th. Would that day work for everyone?

MOTHER: Yes.

THERAPIST: Okay, let's review quickly. We talked about how incredibly serious this illness is and how important it is for everyone in your family to work together to help Jenny battle this "thing." We also talked about the fact that this illness, this thing, is quite separate from Jenny and that our struggle is with the illness and not with her. Finally, we talked about how we, as a team, can begin to make changes that might be helpful for Jenny, and that we will figure that out some more changes when we meet next week for the family meal in my office. Do you have any questions before we end for the day? If not, thank you very much, and I look forward to seeing all four of you next week.

The therapist brings the session to a close, having covered all of the therapeutic interventions outlined for Session 1. She summarized the session and highlight these goals to the family—something she will do every time a session is brought to close. In Chapter 6 we discuss the goals and interventions of the family meal in some detail, before turning to Chapter 7 for Session 2 in action.

CHAPTER 6

Session 2

The Family Meal

The second session involves a family meal. At the end of the first session, the parents were instructed to bring in a meal for their daughter that they felt met the nutritional requirements to help her eat normal and healthy amounts of food. In addition, they were instructed to bring a sweet dessert, or any other item that is usually on the patient's list of forbidden foods. Although our expectation is that most adolescents with BN will eat a more or less normal meal during this session, it is important to make sure that a food item that would usually trigger binge eating and/or heighten the patient's urge to purge be included in the meal that he parents bring to this session.

In the second session the therapist hopes to (1) build on her/his understanding of the patient and family, as well as (2) provide hope that the family can succeed in reestablishing healthy eating habits in their daughter. That is, *the purpose of this session is to join with the family.* It is an opportunity to learn how the family may be "organizing" themselves in relation to the eating disorder—that is, how does the illness affect the family, how do family members respond to their daughter's symptoms, who takes care of meal preparation, do they eat together as a family, and so on. Most important, the purpose of the session helps the therapist to remain *focused on the eating disorder.* As noted, doing so is a considerable challenge in BN given that most patients do not look unwell, as is the case with AN, and many adolescents with BN also present with other psychiatric complaints, such as depression, impulsivity, and substance use, which could take the therapist's focus away from treating the eating disorder.

The assessment of the eating disorder and the family is not a single occurrence; rather, it is a process that began with Session 1 and continues throughout treatment, with deeper understanding of how the eating disorder developed as well as the family's resources to help the adolescent overcome the illness usually achieved along the way. With the family meal, the therapist starts an assessment of the family's transactional patterns around eating and continues to urge the parents to take charge of this area so that their daughter eats healthy amounts of food. More important than persuading the daughter to eat healthy amounts of "normal" food is the challenge of persuading her to eat some of the forbidden food that follows the meal. The aims are to (1) assist the adolescent in resolving any urges to overeat or purge; (2) make sure that the parents appreciate the dilemma the patient finds herself in; and (3) make sure the patient feels supported by her siblings as well as her parents once the ordeal of the meal is out of the way.

The four main goals for Session 2 are:

- To continue the assessment of the family structure and its likely impact on the ability of the parents to successfully reestablish healthy eating in their daughter.
- To provide an opportunity for the parents to experience success in reestablishing healthy eating and curtailing binge-eating and purging behaviors in their daughter.
- To provide the adolescent with the opportunity to covey to her parents the kinds of inner conflicts with which she struggles when she eats a "forbidden" food.
- To assess the family process specifically around eating.

In order to accomplish these goals, the therapist undertakes the following interventions during this session:

1. Examine binge/purge log and weigh the patient.
2. Take a history and observe the family patterns around food preparation, food serving, and family discussions about eating, especially as they relate to the patient.
3. Solicit the adolescent's cooperation in her recovery.
4. Help the parents assist their daughter in eating healthy amounts of food, including "forbidden" foods, and/or help the parents work

out with their daughter how best to go about reestablishing healthy eating.

5. Facilitate supportive alignment between the patient and her siblings.
6. Prepare the family for the next session's meal and closing the session.
7. Conduct end-of-session review and close session.

This chapter provides a detailed review of the steps involved with these seven interventions. The following chapter presents the session in action so that therapists can see more clearly how to carry out these interventions.

Examine Binge/Purge Log and Weigh the Patient

The session begins, as is the case for all sessions in the first two phases of treatment, with the therapist examining a binge/purge report from the patient for the preceding 7 days. In addition, the therapist also weighs the patient. The therapist takes this information back to the family and reconciles the binge/purge count with the parents' impression of events of the week before finalizing the bulimic behavior count. It is primarily this binge/purge frequency log that will set the tone of the session. If the patient is doing well, then the tone will be more optimistic; however, if there is lack of progress in terms of binge eating and purging, then the tone may well be more foreboding. If a patient's weight is unstable or has fluctuated excessively, then this too will be shared with the family.

For a more detailed explanation of *why* and *how* to begin the session by gathering the binge/purge record and the patient's weight, please see Chapter 4, pages 49–50.

Take a History and Observe the Family Patterns around Food Preparation, Food Serving, and Family Discussions about Eating, Especially as They Relate to the Patient

Why

Knowledge of the family structure—that is, the often-repeated patterns of communicating, controlling, nurturing, socializing, forming boundaries, making alliances and coalitions, and solving problems—is gained throughout the family meetings, but may become more obvious during the family meal. The family meal provides strong exposure to the family's characteristic organization. Similarly, an understanding of the significance of the family patterns and the patient's symptoms should contribute to the therapist's effectiveness in producing a change in the way the family responds to the eating disorder. Although symptoms are not believed to be the result of a specific family structure, this does not exclude the fact that there may be patterns of family interaction that render a family powerless in the presence of symptoms. Therefore, a patient with an eating disorder cannot improve until there is a change in his/her relationship to food. In other words, adolescents with BN must regain control over binge eating and purging to get better. *FBT is not effective because it corrects faulty family interactions but rather because it changes the way family members respond to and manage their daughter's eating disorder.*

The assessment of the family is therefore an ongoing process that brings an enriched understanding as treatment progresses. Making generalizations about the interaction patterns in families with a BN offspring—for example, cross-generational problems, poor parental alliances, importance of separation of identity—are at best confusing and at worst probably wrong. For instance, attempts to make Minuchin's description of psychosomatic families as enmeshed, overprotective, rigid, and conflict avoiding (Minuchin et al., 1975; Minuchin, Rosman, & Baker, 1978) operational for both AN and BN in order to produce measurements have largely been unsuccessful (Dare, Eisler, Russell, & Szmukler, 1990; Dare et al., 1994; Le Grange, 2005). These generalizations can be helpful, though, in that they often provide targets for family therapy. The therapeutic meal offers the therapist an opportunity to observe *in vivo* specific family processes, especially as they are brought to the fore during the meal in the therapist's office. The observations gathered from this family meal help the therapist identify unhealthy interaction patterns that might be contributing to the maintenance of pathological eating behaviors. The therapist will use these observations to plan strategies for subsequent intervention. Ultimately, during the succeeding sessions, the therapist wants to disrupt "unproductive alliances"—for example, between the patient and a parent—in order to get the parents to act together in a compelling fashion. Cross-generational alliances (between a parent and a child) instead of interparental alliances (between parents) are counterproductive; for example, when one parent takes a firm, insistent stance, not giving the adolescent any options around eating, or trying to manage the patient's urges to overeat or purge without input from the adolescent, while the other parent becomes an ally of the patient's symptoms in arguing that the strategies are too overwhelming and intrusive for the adolescent.

The aim is to help the adolescent patient set up a meal regimen that would normalize her eating. This regimen would not be too dissimilar from that in a well-functioning inpatient treatment setting for eating disorders. The parents must be coached to solicit the adolescent's collaboration in setting up a culture such that eating and completing a meal occur within a set period of time. The expectation for this structure should be consistent and persistent. In other words, there is no alternative for the patient other than to cooperate with the parents' plan to assist her in getting better. This plan should ensure that the patient does not overeat, either during a regular meal or at other times, and that purging postmeal is all but impossible.

How

First, the therapist should attempt to put the family at ease. The family meal is anxiety provoking for everybody involved, including the therapist. Therefore, an acknowledgment by the therapist that the meal is probably a stressful experience, or that it might be awkward to eat in someone else's office, or that it is strange to eat as a family while a third party does not participate in the eating but talks about them eating, can go some way at putting the family at ease. Second, and in keeping with the preceding, the therapist will instruct the family to proceed in laying out and dishing up the meal. As alluded to before, the therapist does not participate in the meal; instead, he or she learns more about the family style around eating by observing the family ritual and by asking questions about eating. For instance, while the family is putting together their meal, the therapist may ask the person(s) who is dishing up whether the way in which the family is going about their business is typical of the pattern at home, or whether the food they decided to bring is typical of what they might have had at home for lunch or dinner. Or, the therapist will inquire who typically prepares the meals at home, who does the food shopping, and so on. Although this may appear to be empty chatter about mundane things, the reason for this inquiry is quite specific: the therapist is attempting an "inventory" of behaviors or activities that might be helpful to reinforce as strengthening the family's attempt at helping their offspring, or identifying activities that would be less advisable to pursue.

While meeting with the family during the preceding session, the therapist would have made several more general appraisals, assessing the mental state of the patient and the characteristics of all the family members. Throughout the family meal the therapist will observe directly how family members interact around eating in general and around the eating disorder in particular. Here, the therapist should constantly encourage the discovery of new patterns of family interactions by direct instructions and by the way in which she/he addresses the family and constructs this meeting. For instance, the therapist may prevent family members from speaking *for* one another or saying that they know what another family member is thinking or feeling. Instead, the therapist will provide an opportunity for each family member to speak for him/herself or question another as to how she/he may know what the other is thinking.

Help the Parents Assist Their Daughter in Eating Healthy Amounts of Food, Including "Forbidden" Foods, and/or Help the Parents Work Out with Their Daughter How Best to Go about Reestablishing Healthy Eating

Why

The third goal of the family meal is for the therapist to help the parents assist their daughter in eating a healthy meal that *includes* at least one binge-trigger food item. This symbolic act is important, and to achieve this goal, the therapist should allow extra time (approximately 30 minutes) for this part of the session. What makes this session unique is not so much the fact that most adolescents with BN would consume a more or less healthy meal in this situation, but that the consumption of a binge-trigger food provides the parents, perhaps for the first time, the opportunity to appreciate their daughter's struggle around urges to overeat and purge. It also provides the patient and her family with the opportunity to problem-solve strategies to prevent binge eating and purging. For this second part of the family meal, the therapist seldom needs to achieve more than these stated goals, because the effect of success can be striking, and the patient and her parents may begin to realize that they have a new resource in helping her. Thereafter, the parents feel more empowered with the knowledge that they may find it easier to help their daughter eat in healthy ways, and although the struggle may continue for several more months, parental power to enforce healthy food intake alters the relationship among the patient, parents, and food. By allowing the parents to take a more active role in their daughter's recovery, thereby disrupting old and familiar patterns and taking advantage of the family's disorientation in the relatively strange setting of family-based treatment, the therapist hopes to bring about change in the family.

Helping the parents and the patient to address the adolescent's eating difficulties *before* exploring the emotional or psychosocial issues that may be a part of this disorder may seem like putting the proverbial cart before the horse. However, the therapist needs to point out that although an approach that focuses mostly on the emotional aspects associated with this disorder may seem the kindest way to proceed, and perhaps also the best way to minimize conflict, it may not address their daughter's health issues in a timely way. The therapist should consistently suggest to the parents certain steps that they can take to help their daughter eat in a healthy way, including eating moderate amounts of forbidden foods. Similarly, the parents and the adolescent will have to figure out ways to manage her potential urges to purge. In helping the parents achieve these goals, the family structure is indirectly addressed: the therapist reinforces joint parental action, thereby reinforcing the parental subsystem, and begins to "remove" the patient from the parental subsystem by aligning her with her siblings and/or peers. The therapist serves as a consultant to the family, and this authoritative style helps the parents follow his/her guidance.

The parents' first success in helping their daughter eat in healthy ways marks an important turning point for almost all families; typically, the parents feel empowered in that they realize they do have the capacity to begin to defeat the eating disorder. This empowerment also invigorates the parents with energy to continue this task, and the patient may experience a sense of relief that her parents have shown the ability and stamina to help her overcome the demands of the eating disorder. Although the patient's attitudes and beliefs around eating, as well as her relationship with her family, are indirectly explored throughout the first phase of treatment, these issues will receive more direct attention in the second phase of treatment, once consistent and healthy eating has been established. Finally, it is important to point out that the process of reestablishing healthy eating is a joint effort between the parents and their adolescent. The parents, though, are the primary decision makers in this process, and consequently, the therapist should direct most comments about this area to the parental subgroup. Siblings play a different role in this process, which we describe at a later point.

How

The family meal varies greatly because each family brings their unique family mealtime rituals to the session. In our experience most families bring an appropriate meal to the session. However, there are always exceptions; some families may bring a frugal meal for their offspring with BN in keeping with her fear of overeating, while catering appropriately for themselves. Should the latter occur, the therapist may remind the parents:

"You have to help your daughter eat the kinds and amounts of food that will return her eating habits to normal. Giving her this amount or this kind of food [in reference to the portions they brought to the session] will not correct the eating difficulties."

The therapist's task is to help the parents uncover their knowledge of appropriate eating for a growing adolescent, perhaps saying:

"Usually, the best medicine for an eating disorder is three balanced meals and snacks in conjunction with your and your daughter's efforts at finding ways to overcome the urges to overeat or purge."

As is the case with AN, avoidance of confrontation or a quick escalation to conflict in the face of the eating disorder behaviors is often apparent at the outset. However, unlike AN, most adolescents with BN, at least in this setting, seem to eat well. It is therefore seldom necessary for the therapist to do more than ask the parents to sit on either side of the patient and to advise them about how to proceed. The challenge for the therapist is to help the parents convince the adolescent to eat more than she had planned on, especially when such eating will signal to the adolescent that she's had too much, or that the food under question usually triggers binge eating or is on her list of forbidden food. Here, the therapist consistently coaches the parents by making repetitive and insistent suggestions for them to act in unison and to maintain pressure on their daughter to eat that helping of the binge-trigger food item. It is often helpful to remind the parents of a time when their daughter was younger and ill in bed with the flu and they had to make sure that she ate well and/or took her medication. In an attempt to bolster the parents' confidence in this task, the therapist may say:

"Think back to the time when your daughter was sick and in bed and you found a way to help her eat despite her protestations."

or

"You know what to expect from your adolescent when it comes to eating well, and you don't need expert nutritional advice."

While coaching the parents, it is always necessary to acknowledge to the adolescent that this must be difficult for her to have her parents this involved in her decisions around food.

Once the adolescent has managed to eat more than she anticipated or to eat some of the trigger food, the therapist's task is to help her verbalize her thoughts and feelings around overstepping her self-induced food rules. It is important that the therapist helps the adolescent describe to her parents how this "transgression" makes her feel miserable and that she feels like "giving in" and eating more (i.e., bingeing). Moreover, the therapist should help the patient verbalize how overstepping her own food rules makes her feel guilty or bad and that the only way she can cope with these overwhelming feelings of guilt is to purge. This might be the first opportunity for the adolescent to reveal her thoughts and feelings in this area, for which she is embarrassed. It might also be the first opportunity for the parents to begin to appreciate how this illness has impacted their daughter. This new understanding of the illness will come in handy when the parents are encouraged to stay with their daughter so that she does not give in to the urge to leave the room and induce vomiting. This procedure can sometimes be humiliating and even inappropriate, given their daughter's age. However, the therapist's task is to help the parents assist their adolescent in a kind and understanding way and express sympathy toward her for finding herself in this dilemma.

Facilitate Supportive Alignment between the Patient and Her Siblings

Why

Whereas the parents are assigned the task of helping their teenager with the eating disorder, the role of the siblings is different and does not interfere with the parents and their task. The siblings are encouraged to give uncritical support and sympathy to their affected sister; in doing so, the therapist is attempting to establish healthy cross-generational boundaries by aligning the patient with her siblings. That is, by aligning the patient with her siblings, the boundary between siblings, on the one hand, and parents, on the other, becomes less permeable and consequently healthier. This maneuver is deemed necessary if the therapist makes the observation or assumption that the adolescent patient has been co-opted into an alliance with one parent (maintaining a close relationship with one parent that ultimately restricts or excludes the other parent's access to her/his spouse). In such an instance we could hypothesize that the eating disorder would be sustained by this child–parent alliance. The reason the therapist wants to align the patient with her sibling subsystem is clearly described in the work of the Philadelphia Child Guidance Clinic and is also in keeping with what the therapist typically would do in the treatment of an adolescent with AN.

The notion is that the patient will not be able to overcome her eating disorder unless the therapist can succeed in extricating her from her co-opted position in the parental subsystem and "demote" her to her sibling subsystem. This maneuver takes on a slightly different nuance in BN, given the adolescent's developmental status compared to that of the "typical" adolescent with AN. That is, in BN it is generally more likely to find the patient aligned with her siblings, even if this alignment is rather tenuous, and the therapist may not have to work so hard to reinforce healthy boundaries between the siblings and the parents (i.e., clear intergenerational boundaries). The therapist's aim is clear: to get the parents to work together and reinforce healthy intergenerational boundaries between the parental subsystem and the sibling subsystem and, at the same time, reinforce the adolescent's developing of an appropriate support system. In single-child families, the therapist follows these same principles, but the patient may have to find a friend or cousin in whom she can confide.

How

While the therapist is supportive of the joint parental efforts to reestablish healthy eating in the daughter, he/she must simultaneously demonstrate to the patient that he/she understands the patient's predicament—that is, the patient is consumed by an eating disorder, feeling that the therapist has unfairly allowed her parents to insert themselves into her personal affairs, taken away her only sense of identity and power, and left her feeling unsupported as this is going on around her. The therapist may say to the patient (and indirectly to her siblings):

"While your parents are going to make every effort to support you in fighting your illness and help you get your health back, you may think their involvement unwanted and unnecessary. In fact, you may even think that they are being awful to you. If you feel this way, you'd probably want to share this unhappiness with your sibling or friend. You will need to be able to tell someone just how bad things are for you—that is, you will need someone like your brother [sister, school friend] who can listen to your complaints."

Likewise, the therapist will turn to the patient's siblings and encourage them to be supportive of their sister, not in her efforts to be bulimic, but in comforting her when she feels overwhelmed by the turn of events.

End-of-Session Review and Close the Session

Most sessions should end with a positive note, although when there is little progress in gaining control over binge eating and purging, more cautionary reminders may be made in order to keep the family vigilant about the importance of their efforts. It is perhaps nowhere more important to end sessions on an optimistic note than at the time of the family meal. This is usually a stressful meeting and, regardless of the actual outcome, the therapist will do well to congratulate the parents and the family on their efforts. The parents should leave the session with hope and encouragement that they can help their child, and the adolescent should feel invested in her own recovery.

At the end of each meeting the therapist will communicate the findings and expectations to the other team members. In addition to the therapist's impressions of the family meal, below are some of the typical issues that could be reviewed with the treatment and consultation team.

Session 2 Troubleshooting

• *What if the family fails to bring a meal to this meeting?* Failing to bring a meal happens very infrequently but when it does, the therapist should express concern that this may delay the family's effort to address the eating disorder. The therapist probably has two options here; first, she/he can ask the family to explore their food choices in the hospital cafeteria and bring the meal back to the office, or if this is not possible, choose to explore, in a noncritical manner, what prevented them from following the therapist's suggestions from the conclusion of Session 1. If the therapist opts for the second, and perhaps most likely, choice, he/she may have to spend the session reinvigorating the parents in taking on this task and reconvene at Session 3 for the family meal.

• *What if the family provides themselves with healthy portions of food while dishing up a meager or otherwise inappropriate portion for their daughter?* This can happen when the parents acquiesce to the demands of the eating disorder. The therapist will use this opportunity to guide the parents to reassess the caloric value of the portions they want their daughter to eat and will aim to get them to realize that unhealthy or meager portions are not sufficient to bring about a restoration of their daughter's health. That is, not only will good nutrition help their daughter maintain a healthy weight, but it will also make it easier for her to resist urges to overeat and/or purge. Ideally, the therapist will assist both the parents and their daughter, through persistent guidance, to decide together how large a healthy meal would be in order for the adolescent to maintain normal weight without binge eating and purging. If it remains a challenge for the parents to understand or agree on what a healthy meal or regular portions might be, the therapist might suggest serving two meals—one that reflects what the parents believe their daughter *should* eat and another that reflects what they believe she *will* eat. This strategy concretely illustrates the discrepancy between where they are starting and what they need to do to be successful in reestablishing healthy eating for their daughter.

• *What if the parents do not succeed in getting their daughter to eat an appropriate meal?* Again, this does not happen too frequently. However, when this does occur, the therapist should use the opportunity to reinvigorate the parents' efforts to take prompt and persistent action to encourage their daughter to eat once they return home (e.g., make similar efforts to feed their daughter when they sit down for their next meal and prevent her from purging afterwards; cf. Session 3 prescriptions). The therapist will also use this occasion to demonstrate to the parents, once more, how much the illness exerts control over their daughter's behaviors around eating, and that it is really a concerted effort on their part that will alter the status quo. It is likely that the parents will end up feeling discouraged; the therapist could preempt that response by being upbeat in this regard and urging the parents not to feel despondent. For instance, the therapist could say the following:

"You are great parents and have done a really nice job raising your kids until this illness came along. Just look at your other kids and you'll be reminded of your own successes, and there is no reason why you should not also be able to regain your efficacy in helping your daughter."

• *What if parents do not succeed in getting their adolescent to eat any of the trigger foods?* This outcome would be unfortunate because one of the important goals of this family meal is for the parents to succeed in convincing their adolescent to eat the kinds of foods she has typically been avoiding for fear that these will be fattening or will set off a binge. Moreover, succeeding in this task would also allow the therapist to explore with the patient her thoughts and feelings around the issue of having overstepped some self-induced food rules. Eating trigger food items could open a valuable window into how difficult it is for the adolescent to have to deal with these feelings of disappointment, guilt, disgust, etc., and just how hard it is for her to refrain from either just eating the rest of the food and/or the urgent need to get rid of the food via purging. The parents are also robbed of the opportunity to be coached by the therapist to (1) understand some of the tumultuous issues with which their daughter is wrestling, and (2) spend productive, nonpunitive time with their daughter preventing her from leaving the room so soon after a meal in order to prevent her from purging. The therapist is left with having to find examples of binge eating and purge prevention from upcoming weeks to achieve these two goals in a less direct or *in vivo* way.

Most treatment modalities would argue that the initial sessions are crucial in order to establish rapport and a sound therapeutic relationship. This treatment is no different, although injecting a potentially tension-ridden session such as the family meal poses quite a challenge to most therapists. Chapter 7 provides a clear account of Session 2 in action demonstrating the real challenges the therapist faces and the solutions found.

CHAPTER 7

Session 2 in Action

This chapter provides an example of Session 2 in action. It begins with a brief background of the patient and her family. The session is divided into separate parts based on the specific intervention akin to this part of treatment. In addition, explanatory notes are added as the session unfolds to highlight the aims the therapist has in mind.

As a reminder, the four main goals for this session are:

• To continue the assessment of the family structure and its likely impact on the ability of the parents to successfully reestablish healthy eating in their daughter.
• To provide an opportunity for the parents to experience success in reestablishing healthy eating and curtailing binge-eating and purging behaviors in their daughter.
• To provide the adolescent with the opportunity to covey to her parents the kinds of inner conflicts with which she struggles when she eats a "forbidden" food.
• To assess the family process specifically around eating.

In order to accomplish these goals, the therapist undertakes the following interventions during this session:

1. Examine binge/purge log and weigh the patient.
2. Take a history and observe the family patterns around food preparation, food serving, and family discussions about eating, especially as they relate to the patient.

3. Solicit the adolescent's cooperation in her recovery.

4. Help the parents assist their daughter in eating healthy amounts of food, including "forbidden" foods, and/or help the parents work out with their daughter how best to go about reestablishing healthy eating.

5. Facilitate supportive alignment between the patient and her siblings.

6. Prepare the family for the next session's meal and closing the session.

7. Conduct end-of-session review and close session.

Clinical Background

Jenny is a 17-year-old Caucasian female presenting with a diagnosis of BN. Her height is 63 inches, and her weight is 111.5 pounds with a BMI of 19.8. She is currently residing with her parents and younger brother, age 15. She also has an older sister who lives away at college. Jenny's bulimic symptoms began 12 months ago, and she reports binge eating 10 times in the past 4 weeks and purging every other day over the same time period. Jenny does not report using laxatives, diuretics, or diet pills, but she engaged in compensatory exercise approximately once a week over the last month. This exercise includes running and other aerobic activities at least once a day for about 60 minutes at a time. Jenny's exercise served a compensatory function because she felt driven to push herself to burn off the calories she had consumed that day. She reported feeling quite miserable if anything should prevent her from "getting her day's exercise out of the way." Jenny has missed one menstrual cycle in the last 3 months and is not taking oral contraceptives. She denied any functional impairment as a result of her eating disorder.

Examine Binge/Purge Log and Weigh the Patient

The session starts with the therapist walking the patient to her office, where she is weighed and asked to let the therapist know how many times she has binged and purged in the past 7 days. Although the therapist may remind the patient of what a DSM binge is, this is not an academic exercise, and the therapist does not expect the patient to come back the following week with a list of objective versus subjective binge episodes. The therapist is interested in the patient's experience of binge eating and might inquire about the size of a typical binge, but will not spend a great deal of time trying to distinguish between these binge types. The numbers provided by the patient are carefully noted on the therapist's charts and the binge/purge frequencies will be reconciled with the parents later on when they join the session. Although early in the treatment, the therapist still asks with the adolescent how she feels about her progress this past week. This presession time is the only opportunity for the therapist to meet with the adolescent without the rest of her family present. It is therefore a crucial time to cultivate a relationship with the adolescent.

After about 5 or 10 minutes of conversation, the therapist asks the rest of the family to join them in the office. The family brought a meal with them, appropriate for lunch, and the therapist gestures to them to make themselves comfortable and to set out their meal on the table that has been provided.

Take a History and Observe the Family Patterns around Food Preparation, Food Serving, and Family Discussions about Eating, Especially as They Relate to the Patient

THERAPIST: As I told you last time, the reason for this session is for me to see what a typical meal looks like for your family. I realize this is not your home, but it still provides me with an opportunity to see how you as a family interact at mealtimes. I know it might feel a bit strange, like you're on stage or something, but try to do as you normally would do in your home when you have a meal together. I'll also ask questions as we go along. To begin with, I'd like to ask how you usually distribute the food. Do you usually dish the food out or does everyone help themselves?

FATHER: Typically we try to find out who's going to be home or not and on any given night, it might just be Maggie (the mother) and I. And then based on whether people are going to work out or not or have something else, they opt out. And then Peter [son] will say, "What are we having?" and depending on whether or not he likes the sound of it, he'll say, "Oh, I'll just have a pizza"—a frozen pizza or something like that.

THERAPIST: Okay.

MOTHER: All the time.

THERAPIST: Is there much cajoling to have everyone eat the same meal or is it usually . . . ?

FATHER: Almost never does everyone eat the same meal.

THERAPIST: So, it's a little like a restaurant at your house.

FATHER: Yeah, and it's a self-serve restaurant, where people really make their own meals. (*laughing*)

MOTHER: (*asking the therapist*) Do you want to eat?

THERAPIST: Oh, you're very kind, no thank you. I would like to ask you some questions and observe, and it's easier for me to do that without eating.

Some families invite the therapist to eat with them, even though the therapist explicitly stated at the first session that she/he would not participate in the meal. As tempting as it may be at times to join them, the therapist declines politely and reminds the family that her/his ability to observe and learn from them might be compromised if she eats along with them.

MOTHER: And when Mandy's [older sister] home, I'm just so happy because Mandy will eat anything.

THERAPIST: Okay, so Mandy's pretty easy as far as eating is concerned?

MOTHER: Yeah, she's the only one who will eat what I cook.

FATHER: And I eat everything, you know.

MOTHER: Pete [father] eats everything I cook, except if there's anything with cheese or with meat.

FATHER: I'm on a no-fat diet because of high cholesterol, so I'm kind of an extremist. When somebody says there's a problem and you need to cut back, then I just eliminate it completely—that's what I do.

THERAPIST: You told me a little bit about how meals go with Peter and Mandy, but how about Jenny?

MOTHER: Jenny, I don't even bother. Now this is something typical, sort of typical. Jenny and I made this bean dish together. She had seen something similar while we were on vacation and she really liked it, and so she asked if we could make that. So a lot of times she'll make something, but she won't eat a bite.

THERAPIST: So she's a really good cook, but she doesn't eat?

JENNY: Well, I'm not even that really good of a cook.

MOTHER: Yeah.

THERAPIST: Okay, so it sounds typically like when they're hungry, they grab food on their own, or you might prepare certain things that are easy to eat on the go. Is it very rare that you sit around a table together?

MOTHER: Jenny is hardly ever there. Peter, maybe, but he's always on his own time.

THERAPIST: Okay, I get the picture.

MOTHER: And Mandy, when she's home, she'll eat. The other night Jenny went out and Peter and Mandy decided not to go to dinner with us, so they all stayed up there and she sits down and was very pleasant, so sometimes . . .

FATHER: But it's entirely likely that this whole meal would be prepared. Peter might opt out or might just have a variation of it, like just the pasta part, and Jenny won't eat at all. She'll have an apple or something else, and she won't eat this meal.

THERAPIST: So what typically happens, then, when Jenny won't eat the meal?

JENNY: Well, it's because we really don't set the table, so I just don't sit down at all.

MOTHER: Yeah, we've talked about it before where we've said, "Don't eat at the counter," because she likes to eat at the counter.

FATHER: So she'll stand and cut fruit and eat whatever else she's going to eat at the counter in the kitchen. Jenny doesn't often find herself in a position where we all convene for dinner, and there are all these plates and she doesn't put anything on her plate. We just took a 2-week vacation and it happened a lot that we would go to dinner, we would all order, and Jenny would not be hungry.

MOTHER: Well, she'd order a salad with no dressing.

FATHER: Yes, she'd order a salad with no dressing. But there were a few times when she said, "I just ate!", because she would eat something in the car and then we'd stop and she wasn't hungry.

JENNY: Well, that's not a big thing—maybe our schedules are off.

FATHER: Well, it just demonstrated to me that we were all hungry and you weren't.

THERAPIST: This is all very helpful information. Please feel free to go ahead and begin eating the meal you have brought. I'll completely excuse you for eating and talking with your mouths open, it's okay. (*laughter*) Jenny, you're asking your mother to dish the food up for you?

JENNY: Yeah.

THERAPIST: Is that typical?

MOTHER: No, most of the time she will do so herself.

THERAPIST: Okay.

MOTHER: Yes, I say, "Do you want some?" and sometimes she'll say "All right."

THERAPIST: I know you talked about how you wanted to make this pasta dish or this bean dish together. Who usually does the grocery shopping in the family?

JENNY: Actually, I do it a lot. My mom does do it, but a lot of the times I do it.

THERAPIST: How has the grocery list changed after you developed an eating disorder?

JENNY: I don't know.

The family is going about serving themselves the food they had brought along (mostly healthy foods in adequate quantities for all present, including a forbidden food), while the therapist is engaging them in conversation about eating and trying to gather an idea of what this activity is like for them outside the office. A great part of this initial conversation is an effort to help the family feel more at ease with this rather awkward setup of eating in someone else's office. However, it is a valuable opportunity to learn how the family organizes themselves around this important topic—that is, what are the strengths and what are the weaknesses that they bring to the process to address the eating disorder? The therapist will start out by allowing the family most of the time to converse and by taking more of a backseat approach. During this time, though, the therapist takes careful note of what the family does/does not do that might be helpful to Jenny as they move forward. For instance, the therapist has already noted the family's erratic mealtime routine. She may have to bring this lack of routine to the family's attention at the appropriate time and help them make changes that would help Jenny sit down with her family to more regular mealtimes.

THERAPIST: (*to the mother*) When you do the grocery shopping, are there specific requests regarding what to buy? It sounds like your husband is on a low-cholesterol diet, so are there certain things you avoid buying to adhere to his dietary regimen? And what about Jenny?

MOTHER: You know, if my daughter Mandy were here, she would tell you—she's so sick of our family and our goofy eating.

FATHER: But how has the shopping changed?

MOTHER: Well, we shop for everyone. Yesterday we got home from vacation and Peter—now this is unusual—Peter and I went shopping together. He likes to eat sugary cereal and pizza and popsicles; that's his diet.

THERAPIST: Just those three things?

MOTHER: Yeah, he'll actually come with me so he can pick out what he wants. I don't often buy the sugary cereal brand. I get a few other staples. Today I went to Whole Foods.

THERAPIST: Okay.

JENNY: Well, if I get to do the shopping, they make a list and say "Pick this stuff up for us," and I just do it and buy stuff for myself.

MOTHER: But then she'll buy lots of fat-free food for herself, mostly fruit.

FATHER: Yes, lots of fruit.

THERAPIST: (to Jenny) So it sounds like you buy things that you feel comfortable eating so that when it is time for dinner, there will be something that you can eat. Is that right?

JENNY: Yeah.

THERAPIST: Okay.

FATHER: I think that that's part of the reason she shops. She doesn't mind shopping for the rest of us, but she wants to make sure that those few things she wants she does have.

THERAPIST: What would happen if those things that you want weren't on the list? Such as apples?

JENNY: Well, I don't know. Apples really are a staple in my diet, so I don't really know what I'd ever do if I couldn't—when we are on vacation or at restaurants, I try to find the fruit plates and fruit stuff. I never really haven't succeeded in finding apples on the fruit plate.

THERAPIST: What was your eating like before the eating disorder, before you were concerned about your weight or what you ate?

MOTHER: She's always eaten apples. Yeah, but we did eat together.

THERAPIST: So that's the difference?

MOTHER: Yes, and I had a repertoire of meals that I used to prepare for the family.

JENNY: And we all ate the same thing back then. It was like we had five meals that we would always eat. But now it's more complex. It seems like a long time ago, when we would sit down together and there'd always be different things that we ate.

FATHER: Lentil soup.

JENNY: Yeah.

THERAPIST: It sounds like the range of foods that you're comfortable eating has grown increasingly narrow since you developed the eating disorder.

JENNY: Yeah.

THERAPIST: (*to Peter*) Have you noticed the changes in your sister's eating?

This information is helpful because it allows the therapist to see how the family has accommodated the eating disorder. The therapist has noted already that the patient does most of the food shopping, that the parents have allowed her to shop specifically for foods that the eating disorder would allow her to eat, and that the family seldom spends time together around mealtimes. As the therapist makes an attempt to include all family members in this discussion, the patient's brother, who has not been participating in the discussion up until now, is asked what he notices has changed about his sister's eating habits. The therapist also uses this opportunity to spell out the different role of siblings in this treatment and work toward aligning the patient more closely with her brother. At this stage of the session, with the family having brought healthy amounts of nutritious foods for the family meal, the other family members are eating, as one would expect, but Jenny is only picking at the bean dish and the pasta. The therapist is not addressing the patient's slow/little eating this early on; instead, she is trying to learn more about the patient's relationship with her brother and looking for ways in which the brother can be supportive of Jenny at home after mealtimes.

Facilitate Supportive Alignment between the Patient and Her Siblings

PETER: In terms of food?

THERAPIST: Yes, I don't know if you knew what was going on with your sister? That she had an eating disorder called bulimia.

PETER: I don't know.

THERAPIST: You don't know?

JENNY: It's a new thing? Have you not heard?

PETER: I've heard of it before.

JENNY: You've heard of it . . . all right.

THERAPIST: I know it's difficult talking about these things in front of your brother and your parents. The reason why all of you are here is to understand this better and that there are certain roles that your parents will have that are very different from what your role will be, Peter. The goal of this treatment is *to help your sister not feel so sensitive about her eating and for her to eat normally*. As I mentioned, you have a very different role than your parents. As we talked about last time, it's your parents who are going to help Jenny make sure she's eating the appropriate amount of food and not getting rid of her food after she eats or exercising too much. Because this process is going to be very hard on your sister, she's going to need someone to talk to about how maybe she's so irritated at Mom and Dad. For example, she might think, "Why don't they just leave me alone, why do they make me eat a meal?" and so *there needs to be some way in which you can show her that you care about her or that you know this is hard for her*. I think there's some way you could do that, some way that you could convey that you knew what she was going through.

PETER: Should I talk to her?

THERAPIST: That sounds like a good possibility. I treated another family where the brother decided that he would keep his door unlocked and, that way, if his sister needed to come to see him, talk about something, he said, "The door is always open, you can always come in to talk to me," and they wouldn't even talk about the eating disorder—they would do things together like rent a movie or . . . (*Peter makes a face*). That sounds even worse?

PETER: Very unrealistic.

THERAPIST: Really? Jenny, clue me in a little bit on what your relationship is like with your brother.

JENNY: We don't have that much of a relationship, I guess. Even if we did watch a movie together, it wouldn't be like we're really good friends. It would be just sitting and watching a movie.

THERAPIST: Peter, you said it's very unrealistic. Tell me why it's unrealistic.

PETER: Because we don't do that at all. We don't go to each other to talk.

JENNY: Yeah, none of us do. You (*to Peter*) do talk to Mandy sometimes, but rarely.

THERAPIST: Would you like to have the opportunity to talk to him a bit more?

JENNY: Well, I don't think it'd be helpful for me—it wouldn't work.

THERAPIST: (*to Peter*) Are there things you do, though, that are your way of expressing that you care about her? (*long pause*) (*to Jenny*) Perhaps it's easier to try and think of things that would help for him *not* to do.

JENNY: Well, I don't know. If I can tell that he's awake, then it would be like I'm apologizing to him because . . . we fight a lot.

THERAPIST: (to Peter) Well, that's a step in the positive direction, that you're showing your support by not picking an argument with her.

A therapist's task is made easy here if there is already a good relationship between the siblings, and it is not too much of a stretch to imagine how one could be supportive of the affected sibling. In this case, though (which is not that unusual), the therapist has to work a bit harder to find some common ground or way in which Peter can be supportive of Jenny. The therapist cannot force the issue too much either, but has to somehow find a way in which Peter can show his support. That is why she asked Jenny whether there are things that Peter should *not* do, in the hope that his omission of certain behaviors be helpful to her.

Help the Parents Assist Their Daughter in Eating Healthy Amounts of Food, Including "Forbidden" Foods, and/or Help the Parents Work Out with Their Daughter How Best to Go about Reestablishing Healthy Eating

THERAPIST: (turning to Jenny) Jenny, would you feel okay talking about what it's like to sit down at dinner or what it's like sitting here where everyone has been eating the meal? I've noticed that your mom is done eating, and Peter is done eating, and your dad is almost done eating. But I notice that half of your plate is left. Would you feel comfortable telling us what's going on? What goes on when you're at home, and you know it's dinnertime, and you have to eat something?

JENNY: Um, I don't know. I don't actually like to eat full meals, I'd rather snack. I never felt like there was . . . well, maybe I don't feel relaxed.

THERAPIST: Is any part of this not feeling relaxed about your feeling uncomfortable with the amount of calories you're eating, or calculating how many fat grams are in this meal, or . . .

JENNY: Well, I just (pause) . . . I don't know.

MOTHER: Another thing is, Jenny sits at the dinner table a lot, and we come over and eat and she's offended that we're sitting at her table and eating. She especially gets on Peter for those reasons. Peter is trying to be good, in terms of Jenny, that is, but it's just ironic that she's always at the table, and she prefers her eating to be alone.

PETER: I have a question [for Jenny].

THERAPIST: Of course.

PETER: Does eating kind of gross you out because, just in terms of a meal, you don't like the sound of eating or any one watching you eat?

JENNY: Yeah.

THERAPIST: (*turning to the parents, drawing attention to the fact that Jenny has eaten some, but not all, of her meal*) Does this happen at home where there's food left on Jenny's plate?

FATHER: There would be more food.

MOTHER: Well, occasionally I say, "Jenny, try this."

FATHER: I think she was being extremely good because of the nature of this situation, but at home she would say, "No, if I want some I'll take it."

THERAPIST: Okay, in most of the families I've worked with, the eating disorder has a way making everyone afraid of addressing it. When you're confronted with an eating disorder on a daily basis, I could understand how you would prefer not to address it. I can only imagine that it's not a pleasant thing to address, and you'd rather say, "Okay, Jenny, if that's the best that you can do, that's fine." And so now you're in a situation where you need to attack it and make decisions for your daughter regarding food.

MOTHER: Part of that is that Jenny—she researches things. She's almost more informed, she's as informed as I am, and she knows she can put up a pretty good argument as to why this is okay. And then she'll argue with my husband because he doesn't know much about food.

FATHER: Yeah, not much.

MOTHER: So it's kind of a tricky thing. You don't realize that you're being sucked into this. We're kind of key partners in that, but only here . . . not at home.

THERAPIST: What you're coming up against when you're having these battles is the eating disorder. When it comes to issues about eating, you are always going to be at odds with the choices Jenny's eating disorder wants her to make. (*turning to the parents*) So what do both of you honestly think about what Jenny's eating is like now?

MOTHER: Occasionally, she'll eat, she had some of that bean stuff, but . . .

The therapist has been trying to move the focus more toward the fact that Jenny has eaten only some of what was on her plate. She continued to pick at her pasta and bean dish during the first part of the session and then she stopped eating with half of it left on her plate. None of it was a forbidden food, per se, rather, the forbidden part was that she didn't want to eat the whole portion. The parents also brought a yogurt, which was Jenny's forbidden food, half of which she had eaten at the end of the session with parental encouragement. Typically, patients with BN might attempt to restrict their eating, only to "give in" later to physiological urges to eat, which then leads to a binge followed by purging (which is the usually the case for Jenny). Or patients consume a normal-sized meal but adhere to a list of self-imposed food rules, such as no forbidden foods, eating only at certain times of the day, not eating after 10 P.M., and so on. When there is transgression of these rules, patients usually give in to eating unusually large amounts, followed by purging. Either of these presentations could be evident at the family meal. In the case of Jenny, she did not eat a sufficient amount, nor did she eat much of the yogurt, which is what the parents brought from Jenny's self-imposed "forbidden food" list. The therapist's task will be to help the parents convince Jenny to eat a more appropriate meal, which under these circumstances would be to finish her plate of pasta and the bean dish. In other words, the goal is for the parents to support their adolescent to eat what most people would consider a normal amount of food for the occasion. In this case, at lunchtime, the parents were accurate in their conception of a nutritious meal. Most parents need little education around appropriate food choices or amounts of food.

THERAPIST: But are you okay with what she's eaten today? Do you think it's enough for someone her age?

MOTHER: When I think of it, I have a problem when she binges. So if she would eat consistently and have a main group-based diet, I'm okay with that. I'd like her to put something in her salad. And she eats a lot of bread; I think that's a part of your diet.

FATHER: I just don't know enough about it. I . . .

THERAPIST: Let's take your other daughter Mandy, for example. When Mandy was Jenny's age, was her eating different from how Jenny eats?

FATHER: She always had a very hearty appetite, and she might eat even five meals a day. I mean, she's very active. Jenny's very active too, but she complains that she is eating way too much food and that she wishes she could control her appetite a little bit. They are very different.

MOTHER: Mandy doesn't overeat, but Jenny does.

FATHER: She [Mandy] enjoys a good meal, and it's a good thing she's as active as she is. But, for her, I don't see any problem at all. In terms of Jenny, I know she's not eating. I would say, too, I don't know how to address it directly. I want to address it directly.

THERAPIST: So you see that she's eating an apple and that's dinner?

FATHER: We just took a 2-week vacation, and those were all times that we were trapped in the car together and going to all the same events together and coming back to our hotel together. (*turning to Jenny*) You ate nothing those days. I know that on other days you eat a lot more, but are you eating a lot more on those days because you have a lot more private time and so, if you want to, you can purge? So you behave differently, like you know you're going to be with us, and you can't control that, so you behave differently. You just don't eat anything. And it just got me thinking. I don't usually spend that much time with Jenny, so I don't know exactly what she's eating, but I do see when something is supposed to be dinner and it's not food. There are two things about me. I like to address problems head on, and I'm the guy in the family who says, "Don't worry, everything's okay," "*It will all be all right, you'll be happy, everything will be fine*," and I like to lead my life that way. I'm so afraid that by dealing with Jenny and this issue head on, not knowing what I'm doing, I could eventually push her away. Then I wouldn't have helped her, and I know I wouldn't have a relationship with her. So, up to this point, I've opted to have a relationship and nurture the other parts of her, and ignore the bulimic thing, because I really don't know what my role is supposed to be.

THERAPIST: Okay . . . okay, that's exactly why you're here: to find out what your role is (*said with an understanding/supportive tone*).

FATHER: Well, am I happy with the way that she's eating? (*turning to Jenny*) I can't imagine that the amount of food you eat some days could sustain anyone.

MOTHER: When Jenny doesn't eat enough, she gets really grouchy. When she was a baby, she was this way, too. I guess she has low blood sugar, and we knew that if Jenny was grouchy, we just needed to give her something to eat and she'd be fine. And so I judge her on that. If she's in a cheerful mood, I figure she had enough to eat, and I don't look specifically at what she's eating.

THERAPIST: But you both know as her parents how much your daughter ought to be eating to be healthy. A lot of times parents will say, "Can I have a nutritionist tell me exactly what my child should be eating?", and I would say, "Well, certainly you could work with a nutritionist who could provide you with excellent nutritional information, but I really don't believe that parents need to be told what a healthy girl, of your daughter's age, should be eating."

MOTHER: It's tough for Jenny, it's tough because—I feel like I have a healthy diet and if everyone would eat what I eat, I'd be really happy, you know. But it is hard, I have five different people to feed.

THERAPIST: But you know what is an appropriate dinner for Jenny. I think you know that as her parents.

MOTHER: If she ate that (*pointing to what's on Jenny's plate—a medium portion of pasta, a bean dish, both of which she has eaten about 50%*) I'd be thrilled.

THERAPIST: (*to the father*) Do you feel the same way as your wife?

FATHER: Yes, and I think there'd be no lack of ideas on how Jenny could put together three meals and three snacks. I'd think she'd have no problem with it. I think she's doing the three snacks, not all those meals, but if she started putting three meals together, there wouldn't be any problem.

The therapist has helped the parents understand some of the internal dilemmas that Jenny might be feeling in relation to food; that is, she can eat only small amounts when she has no escape to purge. When she's alone and in control, it is easier to eat large amounts of food because purging afterward becomes an option. The therapist's challenge here is to convince the parents to help Jenny eat what is on her plate—which, in her subjective experience, will be too large an amount to be comfortable with and would lead to the urge to induce vomiting. It is important for the parents to succeed in getting Jenny to eat more—including, if possible, a type of food that Jenny normally considers off-limits—but equally important to learn more about their daughter's fears and concerns around eating. This is also a good opportunity for the therapist to turn more attention toward Jenny and sympathize with her, given the unenviable position in which she finds herself. For instance, in the passages to follow, the therapist turns to the patient and sympathetically paraphrases Jenny's likely thoughts in situations where purging would be difficult or embarrassing: "I don't want to be purging, so then everything that I eat will be a little amount or my safe foods because I can't get rid of it."

THERAPIST: You said if she would eat the rest of what's on her plate, you'd be thrilled. So you know what she needs to be eating, but yet you're up against the eating disorder that causes her to eat hardly anything.

FATHER: (*turning to Jenny*) When you came back from Michigan, you looked remarkably thin. I know you had just spent a week with Cathy and Julia. In close company, probably spending most of your time with them, all I can think about is that you just stopped eating because you didn't want to do anything else that might cause embarrassment or awkwardness. So you literally were eating very little. I was a little shocked at how much thinner you looked when you came back.

THERAPIST: (to Jenny) I can see how the illness you have gets you to think this is a solution: "I don't want to be purging, so then I will eat only a little amount or only my safe foods because I can't get rid of it." So I imagine it's pretty scary to sit here and listen to me tell your parents that they know what they should be feeding you and they should not allow you to purge. (to parents) You may think that this strategy is not being respectful of someone Jenny's age. It might be off-putting for you to be this involved in your daughter's eating, who, in every other respect, can make healthy decisions. However, what's going on in your daughter's head, when it comes to decisions about eating and food, is too much to figure out on her own. "Should I have the fat-free yogurt or should I have the carrot sticks? Which one has less fat, I'm not sure, perhaps it's better not to have anything." It just becomes easier to not eat. So in many ways the kindest thing that you can do would be if you both make the decision about what you think would be a healthy breakfast for her, what's a healthy lunch, what's a healthy dinner, what are good snacks, and not allow her to have the opportunity to get rid of these food items. You can expect her not to be happy with you, but remind yourselves that you're not dealing with Jenny, you're confronting the illness. If she didn't have this illness, she wouldn't be fighting you. The eating disorder is stronger than your daughter at this point, and it's making all of her decisions about what it is that she should or should not eat. You have to outsmart the eating disorder, and you're the ones who know how best to accomplish this so that your daughter is healthy again. (to Jenny) Right now, it's too difficult for you to make these choices on your own. I'd like to think there's a part of you, at the end of this treatment, that would say "I'm glad that my parents actually took control over my eating because I couldn't do it at that time." Jenny, I also said last time you have a very valuable role in this, in that I know you don't want these symptoms. Last week I said that we should treat this no differently than if you were diagnosed with cancer. (turning to the parents) I know what both of you would do in such a circumstance: There would be no second-guessing. It would be, "Okay, we need to find the best oncology specialist, and if the oncologist recommends radiation, chemotherapy, we'll make sure that she goes to every appointment—we have to eradicate this tumor. I would say that this bulimia should be no different." Here the tumor is that she has bulimia, and the treatment is that the parents be stronger than this illness. That treatment is going to allow her to make healthy decisions about her eating.

FATHER: I agree. I don't think there's anything that we won't find a way to work on. Then there's the working out, you know, I think Jenny truly enjoys working out, but I can see how that also works hand in hand with, "Well, I ate lunch so I have to work out especially hard."

MOTHER: Because we are so health conscious and she's really into no trans fatty acids and all those things, so . . .

FATHER: So a good hunk of cheese would be interesting!

MOTHER: It just wouldn't sit well with her for several reasons. That's why we just brought yogurt.

THERAPIST: Is that something you wouldn't normally eat?

JENNY: No.

THERAPIST: The reason why we asked you to bring a food that makes Jenny feel uncomfortable or is a "forbidden" food is for us to be confronted with the eating disorder and to provide you both with an opportunity to be stronger than, and in control of, the eating disorder. Both of you should agree on what she should eat and how much she should eat.

MOTHER: Yeah, you know, like I said, if she ate that, then I'd be happy. So I don't quite understand what . . .

FATHER: Maggie . . .

THERAPIST: You decided what it is that you prefer.

FATHER: Maggie and I—Maggie more than myself—often have yogurt and granola and fresh fruit and call that a breakfast.

THERAPIST: Okay.

FATHER: And we both find that completely filling and adequate. It might be that the bowl we prepare is much larger than what Jenny would want to eat, but certainly . . . she eats food that isn't granola. She eats apples and pudding and yogurt, and even though it's fat free, it still possesses some of the things that yogurt has. A moderate-sized bowl for breakfast, to me, seems completely adequate as one kind of a breakfast.

The therapist is becoming a little exasperated with the parents' stalling around the task at hand, which is to get their daughter to eat a little more than she was prepared to eat coming into the session. So the therapist turns to the parents again and points out that they should now try to convince Jenny to eat a bit more, here, in the session.

THERAPIST: What is it that you would like for her to eat now?

FATHER: I don't know.

THERAPIST: How can you both convey to Jenny what you would like her to eat? Is there anything you could say? (*pause*) Could you say, "Jenny, we want you to finish what's on your plate"?

FATHER: Yes, that's what we would say.

THERAPIST: Try saying that now, directly to her.

FATHER: Jenny . . . I'd like you to eat the two different foods there. I'd like you to eat a half portion of each one of those foods.

JENNY: Okay.

FATHER: That's very good.

MOTHER: Can you do it?

THERAPIST: (*to the mother*) Do you agree with your husband?

MOTHER: Yes, I don't see why she should eat all of it.

THERAPIST: Would you be able to back him up?

MOTHER: Yeah, I mean if he asked me to eat that much, I would easily be able to eat that. (*to Jenny*) Your dad was scarfing down . . .

Despite the therapist's efforts to get the parents to agree on the same amount, and to back each other up, they (the parents) are struggling to say and do exactly the same thing. The therapist perseveres, though.

FATHER: . . . despite everyone watching and probably being slightly annoyed.

MOTHER: So, what do you prefer to eat?

JENNY: I don't know. I guess . . .

THERAPIST: May I interrupt? I know that you're just trying to be so respectful of Jenny's feelings and I would be in favor of that if we were discussing any other topic other than eating, but I am trying to get you to address the eating disorder. Keep in mind who you are consulting with. I think that you're thinking you're consulting with Jenny, but you're actually consulting with the bulimia.

MOTHER: Uh-huh.

THERAPIST: And bulimia is always going to answer, "I'm really not hungry," or "I'm not up for it now," or "It looks disgusting." The eating disorder will always try to find a way out of the situation. It would prefer to walk away from the table only having to eat a little bit on the plate. The last thing I want is for you both to walk out of here feeling defeated. You can do this.

Again confronted by the therapist to move forward firmly to help Jenny eat a little more, Mother stalls and diverts the attention to her son Peter. The therapist wants to be respectful of this move, will go along with the parents for a little while, but then bring the discussion back to helping her and her husband work together to help Jenny to eat more. Mother inadvertently provides the therapist with the opportunity to point out Peter's specific role as Jenny's sibling: that of not getting involved in the struggle around eating, because the struggle around food is the parents' domain.

MOTHER: Peter looks a little dazed and confused.

THERAPIST: Peter, remember that you don't have the task that your parents have.

PETER: What's my task then?

THERAPIST: Your task is to . . .

JENNY: Be there.

THERAPIST: Exactly, be supportive.

PETER: So she comes into the basement swearing that Mom and Dad are being cruel and unusual (*laughter*).

FATHER: But I would like to be able to help her, too.

THERAPIST: Is there a way you could do it and include your wife too? I think the eating disorder needs to see that you both share the same opinion, because eating disorders are very good at figuring out, "Oh, Mom's a softy [or Dad's a softy]. I always go to Mom [Dad] when it comes to decisions about eating because she's more likely to cave."

MOTHER: (*to Peter*) You're probably a softy; we have the same issues with you.

PETER: What?

MOTHER: You and your TV, I do the same thing: "Peter, I'd like you to do this now."

THERAPIST: I think what's a little strange probably about this is that I'm asking you to make the decisions for Jenny regarding eating.

MOTHER: Okay, well, if we ask her to eat this now, is that the goal then?

THERAPIST: Yes, exactly.

MOTHER: Well, yes then, I'm sorry, honey, I'm going to ask you to do it now.

THERAPIST: Your husband wanted her to eat a full portion. Do you agree with him?

Both parents are now making a concerted effort to encourage Jenny to eat more. The therapist congratulates them because they're both working toward getting their daughter to eat what they think she ought to be eating at this time. Jenny started to eat some of the noodles on her plate, albeit slowly and cautiously. In the following passages it will become clearer how the parents' perseverance, and making the same demand, finally encourages Jenny to eat everything the parents wanted her to eat.

MOTHER: Okay, okay. That's fine.
FATHER: That's why we're here, to . . .
THERAPIST: That was pretty good, huh?
PETER: Cheers.
FATHER: That was okay.
MOTHER: Okay?
FATHER: Uh-huh.
MOTHER: (to Peter) So, do you think with the evening meal that you might get things done in time to join us?
PETER: Dinner together is best earlier because I have football tryouts.
THERAPIST: How do you think she's doing?
FATHER: She's . . .
PETER: . . . a slow eater.
FATHER: She's . . .
THERAPIST: She's doing it. She's eating what you wanted her to eat.
FATHER: Still she's using the roundabout approach as opposed to filling up on it. I think which you know is a little different . . . now she wishes you would ask her something else. (laughter) Whatever works.
JENNY: Whatever helps make this ordeal easier.
PETER: Can I go use the washroom? Or do I have to stay and eat?
THERAPIST: You can use the washroom. We're probably going to be done in the next 5 minutes.
PETER: Well, as long as it takes . . .
THERAPIST: Okay. I really like Peter's answer. He's getting it. It's true, it is as long as it takes. But if you need to go, you may go.
PETER: Yeah. Wait, no, but then I'm rushing her. I think that she feels rushed. Then she might throw up.
JENNY: Okay.

MOTHER: (to Jenny) And eat a couple of those noodles.

JENNY: I don't like that sauce. I told you that before my bulimia.

FATHER: But the deal is here that you picked up the plate, you agreed to the deal. You have to eat half. Keep going, Jenny.

MOTHER: Jenny's dad mentioned it, and this wasn't even when he knew exactly what was going on. But, you know, it was clear and it was out of control. Not that he knew it was bulimia at the time, but he knew that her weight, something, was off.

FATHER: I have to imagine that bulimia, like any other disease, isn't packed within, isn't streamlined by those big events in your life. Going to college is certainly one of them.

THERAPIST: And you would feel much more comfortable as her parents if she were healthy and ready to go off to college.

FATHER: Absolutely. I mean, like you said, if she had some other disease I wouldn't pack her off for college. I'd make sure she'd stayed home and we could take care of her. I work from home, which I see is an advantage because I don't have to get up in the morning and flee the house to run to my job.

THERAPIST: That is a big advantage.

FATHER: And it's often the case that I will drive these guys to school—or Jenny, she walks quite a bit. (pause, referring to the noodles on her plate) Just put them away, Ash.

JENNY: I know.

FATHER: It is very interesting 'cause when you were a kid, like all kids, it was always, "I don't like this," and you (to the mother) would take the knife, split the food in half, and say, "Then just eat that," and the guys would eat it.

MOTHER: Eat some more. Just one serving more.

FATHER: Your mother and I want you to eat one more.

JENNY: I don't like it, no!

FATHER: Just eat one more noodle.

JENNY: (Does as her parents insist and eats one more noodle.)

MOTHER: You did a great job.

FATHER: Yes, you did a fantastic job!

Although the parents were inclined to get somewhat distracted in their task of relentlessly making sure Jenny ate a reasonable amount at this session, the therapist succeeds at keeping them on task. The parents also show, eventually, a welcome ability to back each other up in their demand that

Jenny eat half of what's on her plate. The parents succeed, and Jenny eats everything they asked her to eat. Understanding that it must have been difficult for Jenny, the parents shower her with praise when the job is done.

End-of-Session Review and Close the Session

THERAPIST: (*to Jenny*) I know this was probably quite difficult for you. The reason why we do this is for me to see what we're up against here. Of course, we can talk about the eating disorder and how it trips you up, but it's quite another thing when you are confronted with the food, and we can really see how much food and eating scares you. We're all here to do this; we're all on your side, and none of us is on bulimia's side. I hope you can see, Jenny, that we're fighting against the eating disorder and not against you. (*to the parents*) I think this was a very important session. You both did a wonderful job of sending her the message that in order to beat an eating disorder, you all have to be stronger, the intervention has to be stronger, than the illness.

MOTHER: So do we get any assignments then?

THERAPIST: The assignment is for you to do what we discussed; the prescription is three meals and in-between snacks per day, and for you both to agree on what is a healthy amount of food for Jenny to eat during each of those meals and snacks.

FATHER: So should we decide what the three meals and three snacks are?

THERAPIST: You can certainly do it like that, but there can also be input from Jenny. I don't want this to be "Jenny, you have no choice." It really should be a collaborative effort from all of you.

FATHER: Yeah, we're not going to ask her to alter her diet outrageously, that's not our motive at all. We're just meaning to encourage her to have a regular meal with us.

THERAPIST: Absolutely. As you learned tonight, whenever you're consulting Jenny about food, you're not consulting with her, but with bulimia. So it may feel, Jenny, a little like I'm unleashing your parents on you. I am unleashing them when it comes to your eating. But I want them to treat you like Jenny in every other respect. Do you have any questions? Thank you for being so patient and, Peter, I'm really glad that you came to the session. Do you have any questions?

PETER: It was fun.

THERAPIST: Was it really? Any questions for me?

PETER: Uh, no, I'm good.

THERAPIST: We should set up an appointment to meet next week at the same time then.

PETER: Wait, no, I do have a question.

THERAPIST: Yes?

PETER: Am I coming back here next week?

THERAPIST: I will leave that up to you and your parents. When you are able to come, I think it would be helpful because you live at home and can give us your perspective on what your sister is going through. But I also understand that it may not be possible for you come to every session. Did that answer your question?

PETER: Absolutely.

FATHER: Great. Thank you.

The therapist did a focused job in keeping the family on track throughout a session that included possible tangents to the task at hand. The therapist identified the family's strengths around eating, learned about the patient's relationship with her brother and how he can be supportive of her while the parents are helping her regain healthy eating habits, and finally, encouraged the parents to convince the patient to eat what is considered an appropriate amount of food, given her age and the occasion. The family succeeded and the therapist could send them off feeling encouraged that they have the tools they need to help Jenny move forward. However, much still has to change in order for Jenny to move clearly away from her eating disorder. The ensuing chapters take the reader through the important tasks for the remainder of the first phase of treatment and provide an example of a typical treatment session toward the end of Phase I.

CHAPTER 8

The Remainder of Phase I
(Sessions 3–10)

The remainder of the first phase of treatment is characterized by the therapist's attempts to assist the parents and the adolescent in bringing most of the patient's food intake under their (parents and adolescent, working together) joint control, which includes strategies to curtail binge-eating and purging behaviors. Expanding, reinforcing, and repeating some of the tasks initiated at the beginning of therapy accomplish this task. What the therapist needs to achieve in Sessions 3–10, in addition to continuing the work begun in Sessions 1 and 2, is to (1) review with the parents, on a regular basis, their attempts at helping their daughter reestablish healthy eating habits, and (2) systematically advise the parents on how to proceed in curtailing the influence of the eating disorder. Sessions are characterized by a considerable degree of repetition; the therapist may go over the same steps week after week to get the parents and the adolescent to become consistent in instituting regular eating and implementing strategies to make sure the adolescent manages not to overeat or purge. Unlike the more structured nature of the first two meetings, the following sessions may seem less systematically organized, and may not follow a prespecified order. However, a combination of the following four goals will apply to almost every session until the conclusion of the first phase of treatment:

- Keep the treatment focused on the eating disorder and manage comorbidities separately.
- Help the parents take charge of reestablishing healthy eating habits.

- Guide parents to employ strategies that curtail binge eating and purging.
- Mobilize siblings to support the patient.

In order to accomplish these goals, the following interventions are appropriate to consider during the remainder of Phase I treatment:

1. Collect binge/purge log and weigh patient at the beginning of each session.
2. Direct, redirect, and focus therapeutic discussion on food and eating behaviors and their management until food eating, and weight behaviors are normalized.
3. Manage an acute problem (e.g., a comorbid issue) and then refocus on BN.
4. Discuss and support parents' efforts at reestablishing healthy eating.
5. Discuss, support, and help family members evaluate efforts of siblings to support their sibling with BN.
6. Continue to modify parental and sibling criticisms.
7. Continue to distinguish the patient and her interests from those of BN.
8. Close all sessions by recounting points of progress.

These interventions will be applied in Sessions 4–10 in any order, with their momentary applicability or appropriateness determined by the family's response to the initial interventions conducted in Sessions 1–3. For the purpose of clarification, however, we outline a description of each intervention separately, even though in practice they may overlap to a considerable degree. Patients may require a range of sessions for completion of Phase I, sometimes as few as two or three additional sessions to as many as 10 or more.

Collect Binge/Purge Log and Weigh the Patient at the Beginning of Each Session

Why

As in the first two sessions, discussing the binge/purge log for the past week and weighing the patient is an important opportunity to assess progress.

Monitoring progress this way is important in the same way that monitoring weight is primary in the treatment of AN. Just as the weight chart sets the tone for the session in AN, the binge/purge log sets the tone for each meeting in BN. It is also an opportunity to continue to build rapport with the patient. Because the parents are being encouraged by the therapist to take an active role in reestablishing healthy eating, at times against the wishes of the adolescent, the remainder of the first phase of treatment could put strain on the relationship between the therapist and the patient. It is therefore of considerable help to be both sympathetic and accessible to the patient during these brief periods of one-on-one interaction. At these check-in periods it is always useful to ask the adolescent specifically whether there are any issues she would like the therapist to put forward in the session. The therapist usually makes a general inquiry as to how the past week has gone. More specifically, the therapist wants to make sure that these few minutes give the adolescent the opportunity to talk about events of the past week that she does not necessarily want her parents to be aware of. For the most part, the therapist will keep this communication in confidence, provided that self-harm or harm to others is not on this list of topics.

Reestablishing healthy eating is usually a variable process. In one family, parents may readily take up the task of helping their daughter and relatively quickly figure out how to establish regular eating and a way to monitor post mealtimes so as to prevent purging. In other families, parents may struggle with a variety of issues that prevent them from being more effective. For example, parents may have trouble working together as a team, they may disagree on the best strategy to employ in preventing binges, or how best to let their daughter know that the bathroom might be off-limits for 40 minutes following mealtimes. One of them may not make it a priority to be present at mealtimes, or both may think it unnecessary to be "this involved" in their child's recovery. Most often, the parents are extremely reluctant to take on the strong will of their child with BN because they know what they are up against and do not want to face this challenge. In some cases, one parent may be overinvolved with the accomplishments of the affected child and be unwilling to challenge her behaviors. For example, one parent desperately wanted her daughter to continue participating on the track team, even though the coach overemphasized "weight guidelines" for "optimal running" and encouraged the athletes to purge, "if necessary." Thus the course of curtailing binge eating and purging may be quite variable. For most cases, though, a pattern that suggests that the parents are beginning to be successful in their efforts should be evident by the fifth or sixth session. If progress is not evident at this point, the therapist should be concerned that the parents and their adolescent are not working together, that some aspects of the interventions are not being implemented by the parents, or one of the types of problems discussed above is getting in the way of progress.

How

The therapist's ability to stay focused on the eating disorder symptoms by collecting the binge/purge log and weighing the patient sends a powerful message to the parents and the adolescent that, for now, this is the focus of treatment. The therapist starts every session by recording the binge/purge frequency for the past week on his/her charts and then weighs the patient. If the adolescent has made progress on these fronts, then the therapist will congratulate her and ask her how she thinks the improvements came about. When there is lack of progress, the therapist will express sympathy and concern and inquire about how the past week has gone and whether anything, in particular, might be making it difficult for the adolescent and her parents to move her forward in this process. Once the therapist and patient join the rest of the family, progress in terms of binge eating and purging should be shared with the parents. Likewise, progress in weight stabilization, or lack thereof, is also shared with the parents. The purpose of sharing this information with the parents is to reconcile the adolescent's report of her bulimic symptoms with the impressions her parents have of how the week has gone. Once the therapist reconciles the adolescent and her parents' reports of events, she/he will either congratulate them when progress has been made or sympathize when there has been none. At this early stage of treatment, the therapist should continue to point out that the patient remains in a vulnerable position as long as she maintains an irregular food intake and how this way of eating maintains the bingeing and purging behavior. Parents often take premature comfort from an initial response from their daughter (eating regularly and not observing bingeing and/or purging) and begin to relax their vigilance. The therapist should be alert to this probability and continue to model his/her concern for the patient's physical and mental state, emphasizing the urgency of their continuing efforts to ensure that their adolescent's eating has indeed been normalized and that abstinence from binge eating and purging are well established.

Direct, Redirect, and Focus Therapeutic Discussion on Food and Eating Behaviors until They Are Normalized

Why

As stated before, the primary challenge for the parents during the first phase of treatment is to engage successfully in the task of reestablishing healthy eating in their daughter. Whereas initially the therapist may have to work hard to convince the parents that their active involvement is required, for the remainder of the first phase of treatment, the therapist has to keep the parents focused on the eating disorder symptoms. Parents may become fatigued or the patient may report a marked reduction in bingeing and purging initially, creating the illusion that the immediate crisis has been removed. Because BN can become intractable and can be wearying to continue to confront, therapists and families alike may be tempted to relax their efforts too soon. Moreover, comorbid problems, whether depression, impulsive behaviors, or self-harming behavior, may also become distracting and allow the parents and/or the therapist to shift the focus away from the eating disorder. It is the therapist's challenge, and job, to keep everyone focused on the eating disorder symptoms and also find a way to address these comorbid symptoms.

Managing BN includes parental regulation of healthy and balanced meals as well as vigilance in the prevention of binge eating and vomiting. The therapist should encourage the patient to eat healthy amounts of food at mealtimes, and guide her in determining how much food may constitute a normal meal and is considered appropriate at any one sitting. The therapist may also have to remind the parents as well as the patient about what constitutes balanced nutrition and healthy portion sizes (this point is discussed more in the following section).

How

The usual reaction to the second session is for the parents to begin to explore how they should exert more control in helping their daughter. However, instant changes in bingeing and purging frequency may not yet be evident. From Session 2 onward, and regardless of weight status, the therapist may provide basic dietary instructions and coach the parents in terms of their skills in reestablishing healthy eating. This is done by eliciting from the family their large, but often unused, store of knowledge about what constitutes healthy and balanced eating suitable for an adolescent, as well as their particular understanding of their child. Parents may have to become inventive and create high-density meals, should their offspring with BN lose weight. Although discussions around weight-loss strategies or dieting, per se, should be discouraged, when they do occur, the aim is to encourage the parents to discuss the value of balanced meals instead of getting locked into unproductive and futile arguments with their daughter about skipping meals or excluding certain forbidden foods from her daily intake. Parents have to reintroduce forbidden or "scary" foods in order to establish a balanced and nutritious intake. Any reference to weight should occur in the overall context of maintaining a weight that the patient's healthy body "knows is right"—that is, a weight that is comfortably maintained through eating three balanced meals and snacks per day. A weight achieved through these means is widely believed to prevent physiological urges for binge eating. The therapist should see healthy weight not in terms of norms that apply broadly to the general population, or in terms of fixed numbers on a scale, but more in terms of a particular patient's weight history and future health maintenance. Because weight is a "moving target" in adolescence, the therapist should refrain from setting a specific target weight. Instead, the goal of having a healthy body should be used to guide the patient toward maintaining a healthy weight, which typically falls between a relatively broad range of numbers. Providing specific numbers or target weights is counterproductive and often serves to reinforce the obsessive or ruminative focus on weight and shape that often plagues these patients.

After the first two sessions, regular meal planning remains a priority for the next several sessions, and the therapist continues to stress the need for regular and dietetically balanced food intake. The therapist has to insist that the parents and their daughter maintain their focus on healthy eating until they are convinced that the patient no longer has any doubts that she can remain free of bulimic behaviors while a part of the parents' household.

It is not uncommon to encourage the parents to serve the patient, at least initially, to help the adolescent learn what quantity of food is appropriate. For example, the parents can show the patient that an appropriate serving size of pasta is roughly the size of a person's hand, or a serving of meat should be about the size of a deck of cards. Many patients would remark that they do not know how to stop once they have started eating and/or feel guilty about eating and that they need to get rid of their meal through purging. This is an opportune time for parental involvement. For instance, parents can be creative in finding ways to help the patient remain constructively engaged after mealtimes to prevent purging. Parents may take turns to go for a leisurely walk with the patient, or sit down to watch a favorite movie on television, or participate in a hobby.

In more severe instances, the therapist may have to suggest that parents resort to more drastic measures, such as accompanying the adolescent to the bathroom (while waiting outside, of course), as nurses on a specialist eating disorders inpatient unit would do. Likewise, parents may have to lock the kitchen cupboards to prevent the patient from binge eating. This effort may also include coming to an agreement as to how to spend time together after a meal (e.g., watching a favorite movie on television), how to monitor bathroom visits, and whether to lock the kitchen cabinets if possible. This may also include visiting local pharmacies to inform them of the possibility that their daughter is abusing laxatives and to ask that they be contacted if she attempts to purchase them. This is one instance where the parents may not want to reveal their precautionary step to their daughter; if the parents warned a pharmacist and told the daughter about it, she might go to a different pharmacy or obtain laxatives some other way. All of these steps at curtailing bulimic behavior should be taken only if necessary and with great caution to emphasize to the patient that none of this is punishment for illness behaviors.

As with the prevention of self-starvation, the aim of the therapist is not so much to prescribe how the parents should proceed. Rather, the aim is to help the parents understand that this is a serious illness, and that they need to find ways that will work for them and their family to prevent their daughter from binge eating and purging. As we have repeatedly alluded to already, an important departure from the treatment for AN is that it is of utmost importance to solicit the cooperation of the adolescent with BN throughout this process. In fact, the parents' job might be made a little easier in that the ego-dystonic nature of BN (many patients do not want to binge and purge and explicitly state that they would like to get better, if they could get a handle on their symptoms) more readily allows the adolescent to let her parents take this active role in her recovery.

Once the binge/purge chart has been explained and discussed, the therapist should carefully review events surrounding eating during the past week. The family's strategies to normalize eating should dominate discussions, especially in the absence of significant symptomatic improvements. The therapist asks each parent, the patient, and her siblings to describe how the past week has been and how they have gone about the task of reestablishing healthy eating. The therapist should discourage broad statements such as "It's been an okay week" or "It was difficult." Instead, the therapist should turn to each family member separately and ask her/him to relay, in great detail, what happened at mealtimes. In the same style of circular questioning outlined previously, check with every family member as to whether that is also the way he/she would describe events. Discrepancies should be pondered, and the therapist should search for clarification. The therapist should be able to construct a clear picture of what happens at mealtimes, after mealtimes, as well as between mealtimes, so that she/he can carefully select those steps the parents and the adolescent have taken that should be reinforced, versus those that should be discouraged. The therapist should use these initial sessions to carefully bolster the parents and the patient in their knowledge of healthy eating, and discourage any behaviors that may impede this process.

Manage an Acute Problem and Then Refocus on BN

Why

In our experience, considerable comorbidity accompanies BN in adolescents. For example, it's not uncommon to work with patients who also present with symptoms of depression, impulsivity, and/or substance abuse. Unlike the case in AN where comorbid conditions, with the exception of acute suicidality, cannot trump self-starvation, continued therapeutic focus on BN could be derailed by a comorbid condition. Whereas appropriate attention should be directed to the comorbid condition in both AN and BN (e.g., another team colleague attends to the depression), it is the relative prominence and frequency of the comorbidity in BN, as opposed to AN, that complicates the therapist's ability to remain focused on the eating disorder in BN. Management of the comorbidity will often be required, and the therapist should consistently evaluate his/her treatment balance between the eating disorder and the comorbid condition(s).

How

The therapist should attempt to retain the primary focus on the BN while also attending to the concomitant depression, substance abuse, or anxiety. Although spending the bulk of the time addressing the eating disorder, the therapist should assess the severity of the comorbid condition so as to decide whether this condition can also be managed within FBT, or whether it warrants treatment outside the confines of this manual. At times, the therapist may have to focus most of her/his efforts on addressing the depression or substance abuse problems, before returning the focus to the BN. If it turns out that the comorbid conditions are too intrusive or severe to prevent the focus from remaining on the BN, the therapist should refer the patient for treatment of the comorbid condition outside FBT. Ideally, another member of the treatment team should provide this treatment.

Discuss and Support Parents' Efforts at Reestablishing Healthy Eating

Why

For the treatment to be effective, the therapist must make sure that the parents work together as a team. This teamwork is one of the most important aspects of the treatment. The parents' success or failure in helping their daughter reestablish healthy eating can often directly be attributed to their ability or inability to work as a team in this process. Because the aim of the therapy is to support the parents in their efforts to care for their adolescent, the ability of the therapist to provide assistance in this process is crucial. At the same time, the therapist may be tempted to "take over" the parental role by directing or overcontrolling the process of reestablishing healthy eating. This hazard should be avoided because the ultimate message of this treatment is that the family, not the therapist, is the major resource for recovery.

How

If the parents differ in how to proceed, the therapist will emphasize that although he/she understands and respects that the parents may have differences of opinion, as many couples have, they cannot afford to differ in how they engage in the process to reestablish healthy eating in their daughter. Consequently, the therapist should exercise vigilance in checking with the parents on a regular basis to make sure that they are "on the same page." In carefully reviewing their efforts at this process, as described above, the therapist will also check with the adolescent and her siblings about how Mom and Dad are doing as a team. The therapist should make a point of addressing the parents as "the authoritative team" to reinforce the fact to them, their daughter, and other children that they are indeed in charge. However, deference should also be extended to the adolescent in her role as collaborator in her parents' efforts to help her overcome her eating disorder. Making decisions jointly as a couple may be uncharted territory for some parents. Reminding the spouses that they should work together and that they should be "on the same page, on the same line, and on the same word, at all times when it comes to their daughter's eating" should be done several times in this early part of treatment.

Discuss, Support, and Help Family Members Evaluate Efforts of Siblings to Support Their Sibling with BN

Why

To reinforce healthy generational boundaries between the parents and their children and to prevent the siblings from interfering with the parents' task, consistent support of the patient by her siblings should be encouraged. Healthy boundaries between the siblings and their parents make the parents' immediate task less difficult and prepares the groundwork for successful resolution of the eating disorder and the launching of a healthy adolescent into young adulthood.

How

Similar to the stated aim for this part of Phase I, the therapist should be consistent in her/his encouragement of the siblings not to interfere with their parents' task but rather support their sister throughout treatment. The therapist might say to the siblings:

> "While your parents make every effort to fight your sister's illness and nourish her back to health, she will think that they are being interfering and she will need to be able to tell someone just how much she does not like to be told what to do. In other words, you guys will have to be there to listen to her complaints."

Realigning the patient with her siblings may be a less arduous process in BN compared to AN, as the eating disorder may generally have caused less isolation of the patient from her siblings or peers than is more typical of AN. Also, compared to AN, extricating the adolescent with BN from an overly close relationship with one or both parents may prove to be less of a challenge because the adolescent's development is usually less compromised and a considerable degree of individuation and/or separation from the parents and an alignment with siblings or peers have often been established in adolescents with BN. Notwithstanding, the therapist should be consistent in monitoring whether the siblings are making an effort to involve their sister in their activities (if appropriate), and whether they have found a way to be supportive of her during this process of parental involvement in her eating. This support will obviously vary depending on the relationship that existed between the siblings prior to the onset of the illness, as well as the age of the patient and that of her siblings. The siblings should be encouraged to be verbally supportive of the patient, and the patient should be given the opportunity to express her irritation or frustration that Mom and Dad are "checking in" on her. In some cases, the adolescent has only one sibling who is much younger than she is, or she is an only child. A younger sibling may not be capable of providing verbal comfort to the patient. However, the therapist could suggest that the younger sibling give his/her sister a couple of hugs every day to reassure her that he/she is trying to be comforting or supportive.

This process is, of course, more complicated when the adolescent does not have any siblings or if the siblings are older and have left home already. The therapist should then take careful note of the relationship the adolescent with BN has with her peers, or may have had prior to the onset of the illness, so that the therapist can help the patient identify suitable social activities outside the family where she can meet and spend time with peers. The aim here is the same as with siblings; that is, for the adolescent to become more aligned with her age group and to feel supported through this period of time. To restate one of our basic points that also applies to AN, the job of the siblings does not overlap with that of the parents; whereas the therapist assists the parents in their efforts to help their adolescent regain healthy eating habits, the role of siblings (or peers) is to provide healthy age-appropriate support and activities outside of the management of the eating disorders.

Continue to Modify Parental Criticisms

Why

Parental criticism of the adolescent and her eating disorder has been shown to have a negative impact on the family's ability to remain in treatment as well as the eventual outcome in treatment. Although this research focuses mainly on patients with AN, our clinical experience has shown that parental criticism is of equal consequence in patients with BN. In fact, given the nature of the symptoms in BN (i.e., binge eating and purging), it is more common and convenient for parents to blame their adolescent for their illness behavior than is ordinarily the case in AN. Consequently, it is of great importance to address this parental criticism, which is likely due either to parental guilt about the eating disorder or to a poor relationship between the adolescent and her parents. During sessions in this part of treatment, the therapist should attempt to absolve the parents from the responsibility of causing the illness by complimenting them as much as possible on the positive aspects of their parenting and by continued efforts to separate the illness from the adolescent.

Some of our own studies (Eisler et al., 2000; Le Grange, Eisler, Dare, & Hodes, 1992; Szmukler et al., 1985) have suggested that children with AN from highly critical families may have a poorer prognosis than those from other types of families. The extent to which this statement is also true for BN is currently being investigated (Hoste & Le Grange, 2006). Our clinical experience with families with an adolescent who has BN indicate that they find themselves in a similar dilemma as the families with an adolescent who has AN. In fact, parents with an offspring with BN may find that the symptoms associated with BN "invite" criticism more than the obviously ill-looking adolescent with AN. Managing highly critical and/or hostile parents in families of adolescents with BN is therefore every bit as much of a priority as it is in AN. We have some data on AN (Le Grange et al., 1992; Eisler et al., 2000) suggesting that such families may require a different form of family therapy: separated family therapy. In this treatment, the same therapist meets with the adolescent and her parents, but separately. Without data to support this direction for BN, we can only recommend as clinically prudent similar solutions for adolescents with BN in very critical families. In fact, we have certainly taken that route in our own clinical work. On the other hand, there is reason to explore ways to manage highly critical families in FBT, as described in this manual. Indeed, we believe that it is possible to work constructively with highly critical families.

How

Modeling uncritical acceptance of the patient by the therapist is a key therapeutic task. This modeling is achieved in part by externalizing the illness—

that is, as previously noted, the therapist must convince the parents that most of the patient's behaviors around binge eating and purging are outside of her control and are primarily the result of her illness. In short, the therapist must consistently point to the fact that the patient cannot be identified with the illness. This separation of the patient and illness will help foster an understanding of the patient's behavior and reduce any parental criticism of her. Changing parents' behavior in this regard can be difficult, and it is more likely that parents of an adolescent with BN will be tempted to respond negatively to behaviors such as bingeing and purging. For instance, some parents may say, in response to bulimic behaviors from their daughter, "She is making it so difficult for us—we make an effort to get the foods she likes and then we catch her trying to throw it in the trash or scoffing it in a couple of minutes"; or "We are desperate now because if we just turn our backs for a second, she'll run off to the bathroom and get rid of it all"; or "I've had it with her—I have to be with her 24 hours a day because if I dare let her out of my sight, she's up and down the stairs exercising or sneaking laxatives into her school bag." By contrast, starvation, as is the case in AN, might be more likely to invite sympathy.

These three examples of parental reaction demonstrate that the bulimic behaviors are identified with the patient—the implicit message is "She purges, therefore she's a bad person." Another way to interpret these passages is that the exasperated parent is saying, "I am trying my best, and just look how deceitful or ungrateful our daughter is." As pointed out before, parental anger or frustration or criticism can have deleterious consequences that undermine the successful resolution of the eating disorder. The therapist can help counteract the impact of comments such as these in several ways. First, and perhaps the most effective way early on in treatment, is to disassociate the illness from the adolescent, and to do so repeatedly, to demonstrate to the parents that (as the therapist might say to the parents):

"We perceive this disorder as having come into your daughter's life and overtaken her feelings, thoughts, and behaviors as far as food, eating, and body weight are concerned. It is the eating disorder that is making your daughter behave in ways that you have not associated with her. I am sure that your daughter is a good child and wouldn't necessarily lie to you or act in deceptive ways, such as vomiting in secret. However, this illness is extremely powerful, and it has overtaken her behaviors in so many ways. It is the bulimia that plays a large role when she has urges to overeat and you see food disappear from your refrigerator, and it is the bulimia that gets her to vomit because her illness makes her feel so guilty and bad about having binged."

Second, in ensuing sessions, the therapist should consistently refer to symptomatic behaviors as "That's the illness," or "It's the bulimia talking," and "I wonder what the healthy part of your daughter may be thinking about" or "I am sure if the healthy part of your daughter was in charge, then . . . " when the therapist wants to draw a clear distinction between these two parts of the struggling adolescent. Third, the therapist should make every effort to correct the parents throughout this part of treatment at every juncture when they say something that, in effect, identifies the illness with the patient, for example:

"I know you are very concerned about your daughter, especially when you see her behave in ways you are shocked by or disapprove of. However, it is important that we remember that it is the bulimia that is in charge, that is influencing her to behave in this way. Therefore, we all have to work very hard to help her diminish the power of this illness so that her healthy part can flourish again."

In guiding the parents through this difficult period, the therapist should remember that families have very different ways of parenting and different circumstances, all of which will influence how this process is worked through.

Continue to Distinguish the Patient and Her Interests from Those of BN

Why

As discussed in Session 1 interventions, it is important that the therapist and the family members keep in mind that they are struggling to combat the effects of BN, *not* the independent thinking and will of a developing adolescent. If the therapist fails to keep this distinction as a focused aspect of the treatment during this phase, then her/his hope for developing an alliance with the patient will be greatly diminished and the patient's resistance to the treatment enhanced. Likewise, it will be increasingly difficult for the parents not to respond to their adolescent as being a "bad" person when she engages in bulimic behaviors, as opposed to ascribing her symptoms to the BN.

How

This intervention is described in some detail in Session 1. As Phase I continues, the therapist may stress the need to recognize that more of the effort of eating is safely being taken up by the healthy part of the patient. This recognition can be fostered by saying something such as the following:

> "It seems to me that your parents report that the healthy part of you has been more 'available' during mealtimes, and as a result, that you've managed to keep your food down, and that you are more interested in fighting back BN yourself."

Alternatively, the therapist might ask:

> "As you have been progressing, you are taking more of your life back. Have you noticed that your thoughts are less preoccupied by food and weight?"

At least part of every session should be devoted to these times of observations, questions, and assessments.

Close All Sessions by Recounting Points of Progress

As was the case for Sessions 1 and 2, the lead therapist should continue to review each treatment session with the rest of the team for the remainder of this phase of treatment. At the end of each session, the following information should be conveyed to the treatment and consultation team: the parents' ability to help the adolescent comply with a regular eating plan; any change in the frequency of binge eating or purging behaviors; changes in weight (if applicable); new diagnostic concerns (e.g., anxiety disorder, depression, suicidality); and overall sense of family progress with illness. Discuss any problems between team members; for example, the medical team not informing parents of progress or concerns.

Common Questions and Troubleshooting for the Remainder of Phase I

• *What kind of detail about how the week progressed should be solicited from the parents?* In the early part of this first phase of treatment, and after the therapist has opened the session with a review of the patient's bingeing and purging (and weight, if the patient is losing weight or presents with large fluctuations in weight), the therapist should always have the parents and the adolescent review, in quite some detail, how the past week has gone. The therapist may say:

> "Could you tell me exactly how things were going for you this week in your attempts to help your daughter eat three healthy meals? In so doing, I want you to tell me very specifically how you worked together, how you made your food decisions, how you involved your adolescent, and how you tried to help her avoid overeating or purging."

The therapist might interrupt the parents frequently in an attempt to gain an exact picture of this process. A parent may say, "We prepared some chicken with vegetables and . . . " and the therapist may interrupt, "Who decided and how did you decide on this specific meal, and how did you guys determine what a healthy portion would be, and . . . ?" The therapist will linger over any inconsistencies and try to clarify any differences between the parents and the adolescent in recollecting the events of the past week. The therapist will take very careful note of the steps the parents took that could be perceived as not being helpful for their daughter. Likewise, the therapist will also want to take note of the steps the parents and the adolescent took that did pay off, and will make sure to praise them and reinforce their efforts. Throughout this process, the therapist reinforces the parents' strengths and parenting skills and encourages them to delve into their own reservoir of knowledge about how to raise their children, in general, and how to help a person who is struggling to find a balance between healthy eating and weight/appearance concerns. It would also be important to hear from the adolescent, as a "minority" partner of sorts, what she thinks about her battle with bulimia. We have mentioned that this treatment is more collaborative than would be the case for AN, and these discussions around weekly planning are exactly the point in time where you would want to solicit the adolescent's collaboration in her recovery. Also, as mentioned before, each family will have to work out a way to assist the daughter in this process that best works for them.

• *What if the parents are not "on the same page" and disagree about the treatment strategies?* If, for example, one parent says that they have taken to putting all food away after dinnertime but the other parent disagrees with this strategy, feeling that their daughter should learn to control food intake with food or snacks sitting around, then the therapist ought to explore this difference in strategy with the parents. It is quite important for the parents to always agree on the elements of the treatment, whether it is about food/snacks sitting around, mealtimes and the amounts to be eaten, strategies to prevent purging, or participation in athletics or any other activity that might interfere with the parents' efforts at helping their daughter. It is only once the parents have established their common ground on these issues that they can present a united front and then be in a solid position to solicit the adolescent's input. Ideally, it would be helpful if the adolescent finds the parents' proposed strategy around snacks sitting around, for instance, helpful and agrees. If the adolescent does not agree, then the parents retain the right to move forward in the best way that they can agree upon.

• *What if bulimic behaviors are curtailed, but do not dissipate completely and progress starts to plateau?* Some patients respond well initially by eating better and engaging in bingeing and purging behaviors less frequently. However, at a certain point—sometimes when parents drop their vigilance because they mistakenly think that the crisis is over—this improvement in symptomatic behaviors is halted. After a while, symptoms may resurface and, in some cases, become cyclical. The therapist should explore what started the resurfacing of symptoms and evaluate steps that can be taken to stop them and prevent them from restarting again. The therapist should also use this opportunity to install a "second crisis" in order to mobilize the parents, once more, to step up their efforts to help their daughter. It is often helpful to note, for example:

"Although it seems as if your daughter might be out of danger, this is not so. If she fails to continue the process of recovery, her bulimic behaviors may become chronic and this may lead to loss of teeth, renal failure, cardiac problems, severe electrolyte disturbances, and even death."

From the patient's point of view, as she has begun to eat in healthier ways and diminished her bulimic symptoms, there may be a sense of loss, but not as notably as is the case for adolescents with AN. As we have noted, BN in adolescents seems far more ego dystonic, and although we should not underestimate this sense of loss, it probably is not as severe as is typically the case for patients with AN, who tend to hang onto their symptoms with a sense of pride and often feel that they and the eating disorder are one and the same.

• *What if the patient's behavior becomes more deceitful?* It is usually very difficult for parents to accept that their daughter engages in deceitful behaviors such as secretly making trips to the bathroom to vomit, or buying and hiding laxatives or diuretics. Earlier in this chapter we mentioned, in detail, the importance of separating the illness from the adolescent. When bulimic behaviors are reported in the session or the family discovers such behaviors for the first time in the session, it actually affords the therapist an ideal opportunity to model a noncritical way of exploring these behaviors. For instance, when a therapist discovers that the patient has been hiding laxatives in her bedroom, he/she can calmly empathize with the patient, saying:

"You must be so afraid of the consequences of binge eating that your illness gets you to resort to such drastic efforts to address your weight concerns. What a terrible struggle this must be for you."

In communications with the rest of the family, the therapist should clearly demonstrate to the patient that the she/he really understands her anxieties and guilt around these issues, as well as show the parents that an angry response is *not* called for, but rather one that commiserates with their daughter. For instance, the therapist can say to the family, while turned to the patient:

"I realized again today just how afraid your daughter is of perceived weight gain that, despite the price involved, she can only see herself hanging onto the bulimia as a way out, and that this illness keeps her so anxious about her weight that it got her to hide laxatives in her bedroom so that she could have a 'way out' of weight gain after eating."

Turning to the parents, the therapist should add,

"Your daughter is clearly in a predicament here, not having much control over these kinds of behaviors, and you will have to figure out a way to help her out here so that we can diminish the power of this illness."

This discourse clearly illustrates how the therapist shows sympathy and understanding toward the patient, while helping the parents channel their frustrations toward the illness, rather than their daughter, and insisting that they establish control over these behaviors.

• *How to manage a meddling team member?* As we have stated earlier, it is very important to assemble a multidisciplinary team for management of the eating disorder. It is also, however, important that the team is "on the same line, on the same page" regarding the adolescent's treatment in the same fashion that this point has been emphasized for the parents. It may sometimes happen that one team member tends to act on his/her own, without regard for the overall plan that the primary therapist has put forward. This is especially the case for colleagues who do not have much experience operating as team members or who have not worked together with one another on prior occasions. It is therefore important for the lead therapist to remind other team members on a regular basis, as indicated before, of the overall treatment goals and philosophy, and how the family has progressed in treatment. Proper communication among team members is therefore as important as the therapist's efforts to get the parents to work together.

• *What about comorbid illness and suicidal or self-injurious behavior?* It is not uncommon for adolescents with BN to become seriously depressed or demonstrate incipient signs of a personality disorder. In fact, comorbidities of this nature are all too common in this patient population. Here are only two possible scenarios that the therapist may encounter, both of which are distressing and often tend to cause greater distress in the parents than did their adolescent's bulimic behavior. The peculiar challenge that the therapist faces is to attend immediately and appropriately to these comorbid conditions, evaluate how these symptoms relate to the eating disorder, and return to a discussion of the BN as soon as it is clinically appropriate and feasible.

1. *Suicidal patients.* Adolescent suicide is a major cause of death among teenagers in the United States. Suicidal behaviors need to be taken seriously and managed as an emergency. It is impossible to continue to focus on eating disorder problems as a cause of morbidity and potential mortality when a patient is actively suicidal. Only after the acute situation of a suicidal behavior has subsided can the family and patient be expected to continue with FBT for BN.

2. *Self-injurious behaviors.* Self-injurious behavior that is nonlethal and not suicidal in intent can also emerge in patients with BN. As is the case with bulimic behaviors (which are also self-injurious), it is important for the therapist not to become derailed by these behaviors. These symptomatic behaviors may have always been a part of the patient's

presentation, or more commonly, emerge as there are increasing challenges
to the disordered eating behaviors by parents or professionals. These types
of behaviors may include cutting or scraping parts of the body, rubbing,
picking, and pulling out hair, pinching, and so forth. None of the behaviors
is itself intended to be life threatening; instead these behaviors are self-
injurious and their aims may be variously described as self-punishing, anxiety relieving, dissociative, or ritualistic. Sometimes these behaviors can
escalate to the point that they become life endangering, but most of the
time they are not. However, they are extremely upsetting for parents and
sometimes for therapists as well. We see these types of behaviors as part of
an overall communication pattern within the family and, like the disordered eating, a substitute for more effective communication. Thus, as long
as these behaviors remain at moderately low levels, we proceed with therapy according to the model described in this book, with a focus on the disordered eating as the behavior mostly likely to cause the greatest harm.
These behaviors may become more of the focus, if they persist, in Phase III,
where some of the underlying conflicts may be explored actively after the
disordered eating has subsided substantially. If these behaviors do indeed
escalate and become a greater hazard than the disordered eating, they may
indeed need to be the focus of treatment.

• *How does parental psychopathology interfere with this therapy?* It
is clear from our presentation so far, that a great deal of commitment and
stamina is required from parents in order to be successful in this treatment.
It is inevitable that some parents may arrive at treatment with their own
difficulties, such as an anxiety or mood disorder, which may potentially
incapacitate them in their efforts to sustain focus and energy in the treatment process. One way in which the therapist can buffer the impact of such
circumstances is to refer that particular parent for individual support. For
instance, when a parent arrives at treatment with a history of depression, it
could be helpful to make sure that another professional has evaluated her/
him for psychotherapy and/or medication support. Another way to proceed
would be to acknowledge that these circumstances can potentially hamper
the parents' efforts at helping their adolescent and to encourage the parents
to work out a way between themselves to support one another. Although
we have stressed at several junctures just how important it is for parents to
work as a team and to agree on their strategies to assist their offspring, this
principle does not necessarily imply that both parents will always be
required to work equally hard at this process. Parents should work out for
themselves, based on how available they are, how best to encourage their

daughter to eat in healthy ways and prevent her from bingeing and purging. It is quite feasible that the healthier parent could relieve the distressed parent from time to time in this process, as long as they are always in agreement about how this tradeoff should be managed between them. Finally, we talked about grandparents earlier on, and they could be helpful in some instances. If grandparents are available and the therapist and parents feel that they could be a good substitute, from time to time, for an unwell or exhausted parent, then arrangements ought to be made to have them (grandparents) help out with the treatment process. See a further discussion of grandparents on page 144.

• *How does the therapist manage highly critical or hostile families?* Our clinical experience has shown that modeling noncritical acceptance of the patient and her symptoms and relentlessly separating the illness from the adolescent with the illness is the most helpful way to deal therapeutically with parental criticism toward the adolescent. In addition to modeling noncritical behavior, the therapist will also not overlook critical comments made toward the patient or to the therapist about the patient, although subtler rebukes of the patient or her symptoms may go unnoticed. It is imperative that the therapist take note of these comments and help the parents to understand that it is the illness that gets their daughter to resist their efforts, to hide food, exercise excessively, make herself vomit, etc. In other words, similar to the earlier strategy of externalizing the illness, the therapist should attempt to help the parents understand that most of the patient's behaviors is outside of her control. This may require considerable composure on the therapist's part.

Once the patient and family have experienced some success, it is important that the therapist identify the impact of criticism on the progress, or lack of progress, that the patient is making. This task requires that the therapist identify the issue of criticism and hostility without becoming critical or hostile him/herself. Often these families are exquisitely sensitive to such criticism; in fact, some families show a history of terminating treatment when prior therapists "called" them on their criticism of the adolescent. Therefore, the therapist should identify these problems without judging the parents and then ask them if they would be willing to explore the problems. The therapist guides the parents through the problem to the core issue of the critical and hostile undercurrent that is impeding further progress.

It is helpful if the circumstance being examined for critical comments is both concrete and circumscribed. For example, the adolescent says she binged and purged several times after an argument with one of her parents.

This specific instance can serve as an example of the impact of the quality of interaction (critical) with this parent. At the same time, the therapist keeps the focus on this instance and does not actively interpret the hostility or criticism as the reason for the bulimic behavior, instead encouraging family members to see the impact of the interaction on the eating behavior. Next, it is important that the therapist ask the family to identify alternative ways in which the hostile interaction could have been handled. Throughout this exchange, the therapist must carefully confront the problem of the criticisms while not becoming critical her/himself.

It may be necessary for the therapist to call upon the less critical parent to assist in the process of working on these issues. As a resource and ally to the more critical parent, the less critical parent can often work with his/her partner on ways to decrease critical comments. In other words, the parents are encouraged to support each other's efforts throughout this difficult process. An overly burdened parent may show exhaustion and frustration by becoming more critical of the patient. Encourage the more energetic and perhaps less critical parent to find ways to support the partner in the difficult task of taking on the illness.

• *Should the grandparents be involved?* Although some families live in close proximity to maternal or/and paternal grandparents, we have come to learn that relatively few adolescents with BN spend significant time with their grandparents, for example, staying with grandparents after school until parents return home from work—a scenario that may be more common among adolescents with AN, who are less independent from their families. The obvious question is if and how grandparents should be engaged in the adolescent's recovery process. Given the developmental status of most adolescents with BN vis-à-vis their peer group, it is seldom appropriate to involve grandparents in the treatment of their grandchild. There are probably two exceptions. First, if the grandparents live with the adolescent patient and her parents, it would be appropriate to first learn from the family how involved the grandparents are in terms of their granddaughter's day-to-day care. If it appears that considerable time is spent in the company of grandparents, then the therapist may want them (the grandparents) to join the family for a session or two. This inclusion of grandparents is especially important when the parents are unable to be available in the way the therapist has outlined in the initial meetings with the family. Mostly, though, the therapist should focus on encouraging the parents in order for treatment to be a collaborative experience between themselves and their daughter.

The second possibility in which grandparents would be involved is the case of a single-parent family, because it is essential to have other responsible adults assist the parent in this potentially exhausting process. In either scenario, the therapist ought to pay close attention to the developmental status of the adolescent and be sure to continue the course of a collaborative approach in treatment—that is, parent, with adolescent, with grandparent in a joint effort to help the adolescent overcome her binge eating and purging. It is therefore clear that the therapist should make a careful evaluation of (1) the time the adolescent normally spends with grandparents, (2) their understanding of the eating disorder and their ability to be as successful as the parent(s) in supervising meals and helping the adolescent in her efforts not to purge, etc., and (3) the level of exhaustion the parents may be experiencing and their need to have someone else rescue them from time to time.

• *What if the therapist becomes exhausted by the parents?* In the same way that the parents may show signs of exhaustion with the treatment process, it is also quite possible for the therapist to become exhausted in the face of no or little progress, especially if she/he has been unable to mobilize the parents or unable to impress upon the parents just how important it is for them to work together as a team. Little can be done to rejuvenate the therapist except to remind him/her of the fact that as much as we would want this treatment to be a relatively brief affair, for some adolescents, BN remains a longer-term struggle, and both the family and the therapist's abilities can be severely tested before a turning point in the eating disorder behavior is reached. It could be helpful for the therapist to remain vigilant toward her/his own frustrations so that they do not spill over into therapy sessions. Regular supervision with a peer could also be helpful in providing the therapist with an opportunity to voice this frustration and discuss how best to proceed with treatment.

In the treatment of eating disorders, perhaps more so than for any other psychiatric disorder, the therapist may experience that his/her work is evaluated in a very concrete way through weekly weight recordings or frequency counts of binge-eating or purging episodes. The therapist may feel that his/her work with the patient and her family is on a kind of visual display with these accounts of symptomatic behavior. It is important that the therapist does not respond to the patient's bulimic symptoms as a personal indictment of treatment failure. Such a response will only undermine the therapist's ability to implement this manualized treatment effectively. In such instances, the therapist should consider how to go about treatment differently to enable the parents to find a solution to their daughter's eating difficulties. In other words, the question to be considered is, "What is impeding the parents in their task of reestablishing healthy eating in their daughter?" Our experience indicates that the families are much more likely to feel that they, or worse, their daughter, are not succeeding in the task, as opposed to blaming the therapist for "incompetence." The families' tendency to be self-critical should, of course, not be used to exonerate the therapist from any incompetence in creating the right treatment environment in which the parents are mobilized to take on the difficult task of addressing their child's BN.

Conclusion of Phase I and Transition to Phase II

Careful scrutiny of the parents' performance as a unified team in reestablishing healthy eating in their daughter, maintenance of a healthy weight and control over bingeing and purging in the patient, support for the patient's dilemma from the parents, and reinforcement of sibling sympathy and understanding for their sister's struggle are the main focus points throughout Sessions 3–10. The first sign of the family's readiness to move to the second phase of treatment may be that anxiety and tension in non-food-related arenas have reduced noticeably. Control over bingeing and purging, however, is the main yardstick by which the therapist assesses the family's readiness to progress to the next phase of treatment. Therefore, only once these objectives have been achieved and the parents feel confident that their adolescent will continue her progress will treatment be taken into Phase II. It is possible that many patients will not require the full 10 sessions to complete this phase, whereas others may continue in this phase a good deal longer.

CHAPTER 9

The Remainder of Phase I in Action

This chapter provides an example of a session in action that would be typical of the remainder of the first phase of treatment. It begins with a brief background of the patient and her family. The session is divided into separate parts, based on the specific intervention akin to this part of treatment. In addition, explanatory notes are added as the session unfolds to highlight the aims the therapist has in mind.

There are four goals for this part of treatment:

- Keep the treatment focused on the eating disorder and manage comorbidities separately.
- Help the parents take charge of reestablishing healthy eating habits.
- Guide parents to employ strategies that curtail binge eating and purging.
- Mobilize siblings to support the patient.

In order to accomplish these goals, the following interventions are appropriate to consider during the remainder of Phase I treatment. Note that it is quite common in this treatment to go back and forth between these interventions, not just between sessions in Phase I, but also within a session.

1. Collect binge/purge logs and weigh patient at the beginning of each session.
2. Direct, redirect, and focus therapeutic discussion on food and

eating behaviors and their management until food, eating, and weight behaviors and concerns are normalized.

3. Manage an acute problem (e.g., a comorbid issue) and then refocus on BN.

4. Discuss and support parents' efforts at reestablishing healthy eating.

5. Discuss, support, and help family members evaluate efforts of siblings to support sibling with BN.

6. Continue to modify parental and sibling criticisms.

7. Continue to distinguish the patient and her interests from those of BN.

8. Close all sessions by recounting points of progress.

Clinical Background

Jill is an 18-year-old Caucasian female presenting with a diagnosis of BN. Her height is 64.25 inches, and her weight is 118 pounds with a BMI of 20.3. She lives at home with her parents. She also has an older brother who lives away at college. Jill presented to the clinic with bulimic symptoms that had begun 5 months ago, and she reports binge eating one time in the past 4 weeks and purging twice over the same time period. Jill does not report using laxatives, diuretics, or diet pills, but she did engage in compensatory exercise approximately once a week over the last month. This exercise includes running and other aerobic exercises for over 2 hours at a time, and she reports feeling compelled to work out to burn off calories. Jill has missed one menstrual cycle in the last 3 months and is not taking oral contraceptives. She denied any functional impairment as a result of her eating disorder. She did not present with a comorbid illness.

Collect Binge/Purge Logs and Weigh the Patient at the Beginning of Each Session

The session starts with the therapist walking the patient to her office where she is weighed and asked how many times she binged and purged in the past 7 days. This patient carefully keeps her own log and shares that information with the therapist, who notes the frequencies on her treatment charts and will later check with the parents for their perspective. Treatment is now well under way, and unlike most AN cases, it is reasonable to expect more of a therapeutic relationship between the adolescent and therapist. Consequently, a relatively longer period of time, approximately 10 minutes, is spent talking with the patient about events of the past week. During this time, the therapist checks how the adolescent feels about her progress this past week and whether there might be any issues she would prefer to discuss before her parents are called in to join the session.

Direct, Redirect, and Focus Therapeutic Discussion on Food and Eating Behaviors until They Are Normalized

THERAPIST: So it's been 2 weeks since we've met.

FATHER: Yes.

THERAPIST: Maybe a good place to start would be to go over Jill's binge and purge log, just to show you that her bingeing and purging remain absent and her weight is pretty much the same, around 122. Have you had a chance to review this?

FATHER: We talked about it for a minute.

THERAPIST: You did?

MOTHER: Yes, we've talked quite a bit. Of course, I keep saying, "Did you fill your log out, did you fill your log out?" Last time I think you were a little bit, "Yes, Mom."

JILL: Well, you asked so many times.

THERAPIST: So, you guys have been more consistent, saying, "You need to fill out your log on a regular basis?"

FATHER: Not me. I haven't, because I just haven't asked her. But a couple of times I asked her [mother] if we had asked her, and then she [mother] asked her.

MOTHER: Well, I think in the beginning we were a little more reluctant to ask her. I don't know why, maybe we didn't want to bring it out. But the last couple of weeks we have been more open to talk about it just to make sure she fills out her log.

THERAPIST: I think we talked last time how that may be a good thing; I know, Mr. Kenny, you were saying, that at the end of the day she would know that she would have to fill that log out and that doing so would be helpful. (*turning to Jill*) And how's that been for you?

JILL: It's been fine.

THERAPIST: So it looks like there are zero binge episodes and zero purges for the entire 2 weeks. To get your consensus here, do you guys agree with that? Or do you have some suspicions about the eating disorder, that it is not allowing Jill to report all binges and purges?

FATHER: I actually don't think this time there were; I think it's pretty accurate.

MOTHER: Yeah, I do too. I think it's accurate. She's been really busy with end of school and being a senior. There have been a lot of activities that have kept us all occupied, like with the prom. That kept her busy.

THERAPIST: Sure.

MOTHER: So I think it's pretty accurate.

THERAPIST: That's great. Were there times when you wanted to and resisted the urge to?

JILL: No.

THERAPIST: There weren't?

JILL: Not really, no.

THERAPIST: Okay, so it sounds like keeping yourself busy was really helpful.

FATHER: I just had a question. When we talked about coming up here, and she said now it was zeros again, and I said that is great, I thought to myself—and I said this to her—I wonder if it was just a, I don't want to call it a fad or a phase, but is it a thing that, when it started, that maybe a lot of the kids in school were starting to do it—"everybody's doing it" kind of thing, just to lose weight—and she's gone through that and maybe she realizes that it is detrimental, and now she's smart enough not to do it, and she's overcome it and knows not to do it. I don't know if that's a scenario that works.

THERAPIST: And what do you think about what your dad is saying?

JILL: Yeah, I don't think people in school were doing it like, "Hey, let's all do it," but . . .

FATHER: Have you asked any of the girls whether they . . . ?

JILL: No, I would never ask that.

FATHER: And I wonder if it was, like, girls get together and one girl says, "Hey, I've been doing this to keep my weight down." And the next person says, "Maybe I'll do that," and the next thing maybe there is a percentage of girls all trying that particular way to keep their weight down.

THERAPIST: As if maybe there's a contagion effect?

FATHER: Yes, and after a point, when they realize—I don't care about them—but when Jill realizes the damage that it can do, she's smart enough to know, "I'm not going to do it anymore," and all of a sudden she's smart enough to say, "I'm not going to do it, period." That little guy, bulimia, you said he's still going to be there, but maybe he's smaller than I thought.

THERAPIST: Yes, I think you said that very eloquently. He's still going to be there, especially during times of stress he's going to rear his ugly little head. Even though it sounds like the detrimental side effects from bulimia hit home, Jill—and I think a lot of this even happened before treatment, as you thought about wanting to go off to college and focus your energy there and not have the eating disorder around, needing to get rid of it now—it can still be very sneaky and can creep up on you. I think it's wonderful that you haven't had any binges or purge episodes, but I also think that there's still an eating disorder that's present. That's where you guys come in (*turning to the parents*), to really help, so there's no opportunity for her to follow the eating disorder's path. I thought we could talk about that: what you guys have done as a couple to help Jill, to minimize any opportunity she would have to get rid of food. Could you talk about the food issue that we talked about last time, the forbidden foods, the ones that are more difficult?

MOTHER: Well, you know, in the beginning we did a lot of activities. I thought, with the intensity of the bulimia in the beginning, we really needed to be gone and out of the house for a couple of hours to do things. Then I started taking her to the grocery store with me so we could choose foods together. We minimize that activity now, but I think we're always conscious of engaging her productively. For example, the last few nights I've said, "Do you want to take a walk with me," because sometimes I walk at night, and she'll come. She doesn't like to walk, so she'll rollerblade. Now we're focused more on a role of exercising instead of trying to get her mind off what she is doing. But, as I said last time, I do go to the store, and I'm still conscious of buying foods. I think I shouldn't buy certain foods, but then I've always thought she needs to learn how to have those foods around, and I think she has. The last time I went to the store I did buy cookies.

FATHER: Yes, she did—the cookies have been in their little spot. They haven't moved, except when I move them out. I mean, they are still in the same area. We still keep cookies in the same area.

MOTHER: I did notice that. Those are the things I think we do notice. I've put the cookies in the cabinet, and we could see them diminishing but . . .

FATHER: . . . minimally.

MOTHER: Yes, minimally, over a week, whereas there were a couple of times when only 1 or 2 days had gone by and the cookies would be gone, and I wondered whether . . .

THERAPIST: You'd be suspicious, thinking, "I wonder where all the cookies have gone," "I wonder if the eating disorder . . . ?"

MOTHER: Exactly.

THERAPIST: Kind of, who took the cookies?

MOTHER: But I definitely, in the last 2 weeks, have seen that they haven't been gone. Or, if they have been gone, it was . . . (*pointing to her husband*).

THERAPIST: No, no worries about that (*trying to make Dad feel okay because he seemed embarrassed when Mother pointed to him as the one who "ate the cookies"*).

Discuss and Support Parents' Efforts
at Reestablishing Healthy Eating

THERAPIST: (*to Jill*) Well, I wanted to touch base on the issue of trigger foods, because last week we talked quite a bit about how all of you should not bring these foods into the house because they can be challenging trigger foods for Jill. When we left last week, you felt irritated, like "Why can't we just bring those foods into the house?" I wondered how, during the last two weeks, you felt when your mother brought you to the grocery store, if there was part of you, the eating disorder side of you, that said, "*No, don't bring those foods into the house. Why don't we just have carrots or celery—things that feel safer?*"

JILL: No, it didn't really bother me.

MOTHER: But you haven't been . . . remember, 2 months ago, I would buy ice cream, and every night I would see her eat ice cream. Well, we all have a thing for ice cream. Or I'll buy ice cream bars, and, again, I'll think, "Okay, we should buy some things," and I don't buy a lot, but I'll buy a little thing of ice cream or cookies and we've had that same pack. I bought a pack of those little thin ice cream bars, and I think we've had the same pack for about a month. Well, you (*to the father*) had one last night.

FATHER: I had one.

MOTHER: And I had one. So I can really see that the food is there, and she's not bingeing on it. She may be having a little.

THERAPIST: (*to Jill*) And that's what I want you to eat, so there's an opportunity for your parents to help you eat that kind of food in moderation.

JILL: I can do it on my own.

THERAPIST: You can do it on your own? Okay, well, let's talk about one of those times when you have an ice cream bar.

JILL: I had an ice cream bar last night.

MOTHER: Did you?

JILL: After dinner, yeah, when you guys were at dinner.

MOTHER: Okay.

FATHER: Have you ever had two or three at one time?

JILL: No.

FATHER: Me, neither.

THERAPIST: You have that in common (*jokingly*).

FATHER: I also wondered, we always talk about binge/purge, binge/purge. If you did binge, you might think, "I ate it, I'm not going to purge but I've got it in me, so I'll exercise it out."

THERAPIST: I definitely want to bring that up. I know, Mrs. Kenny, that you also were saying that you thought the exercise was starting to take on a role of getting rid of the calories. Is that what I'm hearing?

MOTHER: No, I don't think so.

THERAPIST: No? Okay.

MOTHER: I think that we are a family that does exercise. Well, I would think that most American families have exercise. So I don't know that it's taking on that role. I just know, in the beginning, when I would exercise, I normally wouldn't ask her to go with me. In the last couple of months, I have said, "Do you want to walk, do you want to go?" Again, she doesn't go as a substitute for purging, but I think she goes to get away from her illness.

THERAPIST: Okay. (*turning to Jill*) I was just wondering if the eating disorder was getting you to think, "Well, I'm not going to purge anymore, but I am going to get rid of the food another way"?

JILL: Oh, no, I like to rollerblade.

MOTHER: No . . .

THERAPIST: Okay, so it's fun? So that shifted a bit for you? Because I know back when you did the assessment with our assessor, you were talking about how you played softball because it used to be that you really enjoyed it and you did it for the sake of the team, and then it was more focused on the calories—"How many calories did I burn?" So that felt different?

JILL: Yeah, I mean . . .

MOTHER: Well, that's definitely different. I think in January and February it was like every day when you would go to John's house and lift weights, remember?

JILL: Yeah.

MOTHER: That's when I think the illness was pretty predominant. I wasn't aware that she was exercising a lot, but I think that was when she was in that frame of mind that "I have to get rid of the calories." I suppose I'm thinking that she is a girl who will exercise anyway, just to be healthy and keep her weight down. But that's not a bad thing, you know?

THERAPIST: When you say keep your weight down, what do you mean by that?

MOTHER: Well, again, I feel that I need to exercise to stay healthy and keep my weight down. I think that's okay.

THERAPIST: I wonder if you guys [the parents] have talked about what weight you'd be comfortable with for Jill and what you'd [Jill] be comfortable with?

MOTHER: Well, we talked in the beginning, remember?

JILL: A long time ago?

MOTHER: When this all started, and we went to that first doctor, she was 116 pounds. I remember the doctor saying that when she had been in before—I think it was in the fall or the spring—and she was 126 or 125, and I hadn't realized that she'd lost 10 pounds. That really worried me and I asked her, "Do you think you're fat?" You did, even at that weight, do you remember?

JILL: Yeah.

MOTHER: But I don't think she's feeling that way any more.

JILL: No.

MOTHER: I was worried because she did gain the 4 or 5 pounds back that she probably needed to, and she seemed to be very comfortable.

Continue to Distinguish the Patient and Her Interests from Those of BN

Mother tends to talk for Jill, and the therapist needed to check with the adolescent to see whether she feels the way her mother portrays her as feeling. It would be important, especially at this juncture in treatment, to allow the adolescent to have a voice and to check in with her about how she feels things are moving along for her.

THERAPIST: This is all resonating with you at the moment?

JILL: Yeah.

THERAPIST: Sometimes I know people with bulimia are very reluctant to give up their symptoms, even though they know they are detrimental, because they are so afraid that they're going to gain an inordinate amount of weight. Even though they know all these symptoms are dangerous for them, they like the effect of the symptoms in keeping them at a certain weight. Really, what we're trying to do, with your help, is to normalize your eating so there aren't any gaps in your day and there aren't foods that you can't eat in moderation. That's really the goal. Whatever the weight ends up being is what it should be, because you are eating a normal amount of food and you're eating foods with fats and sugars in them, in moderation.

MOTHER: Sometimes I think that maybe part of the problem is that she's always done after-school activities, and she'd have lunch at 11:30 or 12.

JILL: 12:30.

MOTHER: And she would have activities until 5:30 or 6 in the evening and be starving, which is understandable if you haven't had a snack. And she also wasn't eating lunch. She was on a cereal kick where she would eat cereal.

JILL: I like cereal.

MOTHER: She does like cereal. Both of my kids love cereal. But I think that that didn't help. When she got home at 6 o'clock, she was starving. So one of the things that we also did, when the bulimia started, is that I began packing her snacks. Before she would go to practice, either softball or cheerleading, she would take extra snacks like carrots or celery, or she would take an apple. Even now with softball, if she's got an away game and won't be home until 7 or 7:30, I will pack her an extra lunch. So I think she's learned that she needs to eat, even if it is little snack, throughout the day.

THERAPIST: It sounds like you have been helpful in that, in packing snacking for her.

MOTHER: Her carrots and her celery.

FATHER: Now in another week she's out of school, which means she'll be home all day. So what do we do? Do we make sure she eats in moderation all day long, like little meals, or do we . . . ?

THERAPIST: I know in this treatment, sometimes parents think, "Well, we came here for you to tell us exactly what to do or to set us up with a nutritionist." But you guys know best. You're the expert on this. You have done a fine job with Patrick.

FATHER: If she's out of school, she's going to get up at her usual, say 10, and then she's going to have her little breakfast, and then we need to talk so that we'll know between breakfast and whenever (*to Jill*) you need to eat something—something that will stay with you, cookies won't stay with you—something so that (*to therapist*) she is eating, whereas before she was going off to school where she couldn't eat.

MOTHER: Well, I may not be around for the first couple of weeks of vacation. I'll be working into mid June so she'll be home alone during the day.

THERAPIST: So, how can we problem-solve this? I'm glad you brought up this matter of vacation because Jill's circumstances will be different. School is very structured. Certainly (*to Jill*) you'll be in college soon and that will be structured, but not as structured as high school. High school is pretty structured. In college, if you don't want any morning classes, you can schedule all your classes in the afternoon or have all morning classes and not have afternoon classes. I think this will be a nice opportunity for you to have experience in creating some structure when there isn't any.

FATHER: That's what I was thinking too. Say, whatever time you eat your breakfast that day, then you'd say, "Three hours later I'll eat something of value." So if you eat at 10, around 1 o'clock you plan on eating an apple, and so you're eating something that's nutritious versus saying, "I'm not going to eat now," and all of a sudden it's 5 o'clock, and you eat something that's not good, thinking, "Okay, now I'm going to eat five cookies." If you structured your eating throughout the day, I would think that would take away the temptation of eating six cookies. One, you're not going to be as stressed and you won't want to eat six cookies. You're not going to be that hungry if you ate the right foods throughout the day.

THERAPIST: When I heard you mention an apple, did you mean that just the apple would be the lunch? Or would that be the snack?

FATHER: I don't know if she eats lunch.

THERAPIST: I see. So at this time . . .

FATHER: So now that you're out of high school, are you going to actually go with your girlfriends to Taco Bell?

JILL: Subway.

FATHER: . . . or Subway. You eat a sandwich, great. But if you don't eat . . . when you're out, make sure you eat a lunch everyday.

Throughout this section the parents are very reasonable in their expectations of Jill and how she can continue to make healthy changes in her routine and food intake. Both parents were remarkably noncritical in their analyses of weekly events and were good at brainstorming together and helping Jill come up with practical solutions regarding healthy eating. The parents were also good at being involved in helping Jill shape her eating behavior but appropriately staying some distance from her other activities, such as softball our going out with girlfriends.

Direct, Redirect, and Focus Therapeutic Discussion on Food and Eating Behaviors until They Are Normalized

THERAPIST: Certainly when you look at this sheet and there are zeros across the board for the past 2 weeks, that's wonderful, and that's due to your [the parents] conjoint efforts. Jill, also, you're learning to beat this thing and not have any binges or purges. I think also you're putting a lot of trust in having beaten the eating disorder, thinking that it no longer exists. But it's an opportunity for when you guys aren't there, to help make sure she has the lunch. I think what we really need to do is problem-solve about how to ensure that you guys know you're helping Jill to have the lunch. There will be times, even perhaps most of the days, when Jill thinks, "I want to go to Subway with my friends and have a lunch." But there may be days when the eating disorder side of her will make her think "Oh, skip the lunch, you don't need the lunch, you'll just gain weight, so don't go with your friends, just stay home and don't eat anything." Then it may happen that later on, at the end of the day, as your dad was saying, you may eat a lot of the different foods that you haven't let yourself eat. I know Jill, this may not sound like an attractive option when you are at home for the summer and just want to have free time, but how about meeting your mom for lunch? I know it may be difficult with your work schedules, but would it be possible?

JILL: No, I mean I'll have a million things to do. I don't plan on sitting around at home and watching TV. I'll always have things to do.

MOTHER: Yes, and the other end of it is that I see this summer—and not that I'm disagreeing with you—but I see the summer as a time where she has to learn to be by herself and to pick her own foods.

THERAPIST: I agree.

MOTHER: I'm worried. I still remember our visit to Massachusetts, in the dorm, and you should have seen this food court. That concerns me:

that she's going to be confronted with a dessert section the size of this room! I'm concerned, I want her to be able to go to this court two or three times and to choose foods wisely.

THERAPIST: I think that is definitely the goal, and I'm sure, Jill, you feel the same way, but I think we still have a few more weeks with you guys helping her before we can move into that scenario. I think that is the goal before she goes off to school: that she has had the opportunity to have her own lunch, or whatnot, but right now I think we are still in the earlier phases even though there's zero binge and purge episodes. I just want there to be more structure put in place.

FATHER: Then maybe, instead of just the binges and purges, at dinnertime we could say, "Did you have two meals today, being breakfast and lunch?" Even if the lunch was just an apple, it was lunch and maybe an apple is not enough, but even at dinnertime we could say, "How many meals did you have?"

THERAPIST: *(to Jill)* How about you, do you think an apple is enough? Would that sustain you?

MOTHER: *(cutting in)* No, I don't.

FATHER: See, I go all day without eating. I go all day and then, when I get done at night, I eat all at once.

THERAPIST: Oh, I see.

MOTHER: What we're thinking of is, if she doesn't get up until 10:30 or 11, she'll have her breakfast, and she does eat breakfast. She'll eat a bowl of cereal or a muffin or maybe some coffee cake if I bought some. So by that time it is already 11:30, so what is lunch then? Maybe 3 or 3:30. But then we're probably going to have dinner by 5 or 6. I actually find myself doing this during the summer: I don't eat lunch because in the summer I'll be up at 9 or 9:30. I'm not saying that we never eat lunch, because we do. Some days we'll have lunch. We'll throw hotdogs on the grill or tacos or whatever. We do eat lunch during the weekend sometimes, but . . .

THERAPIST: Well, I think what I'm hearing from you is that there is not a heavy lunch, or lunch is kind of smaller meal and dinner is more of a bigger meal, and that's fine, every family has their different ways. Some people have more of a meal midday, and others have dinner.

MOTHER: Yes, it's more of a time frame.

THERAPIST: Let's think about that. How can she still have a breakfast, a lunch, and a dinner, and actually some snacks, along the way, trying to take into account your family structure and how that works? So dinner is usually around 5 or 6?

FATHER: The summer is usually later because . . .

JILL: 7 or 8.

FATHER: Yes, because it's still light out.

THERAPIST: Okay, that seems to help then, because you could have a lunch around 3.

MOTHER: I wonder if she wrote it down—is that what you're thinking? That we need a way to monitor what she is eating? To know if she's eating too little or too much?

THERAPIST: You want to make sure she is eating a lunch that you think would be an appropriate amount for her age.

FATHER: I think it would be a bad idea because you're going to have the same tendency to say, "Oh, I'll write it down at the end of the week," so you're not going to write it down. You're not going to remember. I think it would be a lot easier to say her goal is to make sure she eats three meals a day.

JILL: I'll eat when I'm hungry and enough food should . . .

FATHER: Yes, and before she goes to bed at night, we can ask her, "Well, how'd you do today eating wise?" And she can say, "Well, I had breakfast, I had a snack, but I didn't have lunch, and we had this for dinner," and just talk about it. Talking is going to help, too, at night, because when she's at the beach all day, she's not going to be writing it down. So by writing it down you're going to be missing too much because you're actually *not* going to be writing it down. Whereas at night, we can just talk, not say, "Did you binge or did you purge," but say, "Did you eat?" And if she says that she didn't have breakfast or lunch, and just had one meal, then we can say, "Well, tomorrow the goal is to have three meals," plus you can snack.

THERAPIST: I bet Jill would definitely do that. She would want to be able to have those three meals and tell you accurately, but I think this illness really is just so sneaky, and it trips you up. It's especially typical that it can creep up on you. I think it is especially difficult because it affects individuals like Jill who are hard working and conscientious, and there's been no reason to not believe anything she would say, because she is an honest person from your descriptions of her and from the assessment. But an eating disorder really will get her to maybe conceal or not reveal what happened that day. So perhaps, if she didn't have lunch because the eating disorder said "Don't have lunch," or maybe it wasn't convenient that day because she had a lot of things to do, then it could be very challenging, at the end of the day, to tell you because she doesn't want to disappoint, and she may feel ashamed about that, or she doesn't want you to think she's not getting better. The eating disorder gets her to do those things. If I knew the eating disorder was completely eradicated and there was some magic bullet that we could give, then I think that would be fine, but I do think we need to figure out a way that you, Jill feel comfortable with this collaboration between all of us here, where you guys can be assured that she is having a lunch, and, Jill, you're not going to feel like you're in prison.

MOTHER: The reason why, I guess, part of me worries when I think of the summer coming is that I think the critical time for her is going to be at night, because that's when she binges. Also on the weekends she goes out and then comes home, and that's when she had her binge episodes, after I went to bed, so that seems to me like a critical time. It's not that I'm not concerned about her eating lunch, but how will our monitoring of her lunch time or making sure she has lunch help?

THERAPIST: I see what you're saying. Maybe, Mr. Kenny, you're an appropriate person to talk to about this one, because your pattern is that you don't really eat much during the day and you eat more in the evening. But I bet if there is a day when you have breakfast or lunch, you eat less during the evening because you've had that regular food intake throughout the day. So the idea with the lunch is that you're normalizing her eating so that it's really just physiologically impossible to approach the next meal feeling ravenous.

MOTHER: That makes sense. Okay, that's a good point. I understand that.

THERAPIST: Does that make sense?

FATHER: Yeah.

THERAPIST: But I also want to address her issue in the evening, because that sounds like a danger.

MOTHER: I would think the evening would be the problem, but, again, it was after I went to bed. I tried to stay up.

JILL: Yeah (*giggling*).

THERAPIST: Sure, because no one's around, and it's a prime time for her to be vulnerable to give in to urges to binge.

FATHER: Well, my problem is that if she came in at 11 o'clock, and this guy came out . . .

THERAPIST: You keep calling it "this guy," and I like "this guy," not "the eating disorder."

FATHER: This guy came out [in reference to the eating disorder]. If she ate something that I consider more nutritious, like carrots versus cookies . . . she could eat 10 carrots to get this guy to go back, whereas the cookies, it would take her 10 cookies to get this guy go back in? Don't you think if somehow she could say to herself, "If I eat a good amount of good food, this guy won't come out it would help?

JILL: I'll just have carrots when I go home.

FATHER: Yeah, don't you think that the carrots may . . . ?

JILL: Yeah, I think that's a really good idea.

FATHER: Even if she ate 10 carrots, I don't think this guy would say, "go purge 10 carrots," but I think this guy would say, "go purge 10 cookies."

JILL: I think that's a good idea.

MOTHER: I think that's a good idea, but I guess I'm laughing because I'm wondering if she would do that.

JILL: I could do that.

MOTHER: I guess she would want to do the cookies, and the guy might make her want to do the cookies.

JILL: No, I could do that, eat something nutritious. But I guess I'm only thinking of the carrots . . .

FATHER: Well, we could play tricks before we went to bed. If we were going to go to bed and she was going to be out late, we could move the cookies and put a little note. There's nothing wrong with her coming in late at night and having something healthy before she goes to bed.

THERAPIST: Sure.

FATHER: Or some celery. I think that would be good.

JILL: That'd be good.

THERAPIST: Yeah, I just want to make sure, Jill, that you have this guy under control, because I've heard now that your parents are concerned about your going off to college where there's this food court that I'm sure is magnified in their minds times 10.

MOTHER: Well, it is.

FATHER: This Willy Wonka structure.

MOTHER: You should have seen it though, remember? That dessert room?

THERAPIST: (to Jill) I think what I'm hearing, correct me if I'm wrong, is that they want you to have experience with eating these foods. And they're not bad foods. There are no bad foods. Certainly it's the amount that you eat of them. (*to the parents*) And I definitely like what you were saying. You want to make sure that your daughter is eating nutritionally, just like you want Patrick [Jill's brother] to make sure he's getting enough minerals and proteins and fats, all of those things. I would think you'd want her to have some experience with eating some cookies and eating ice cream, not having three bowls of ice cream, but one bowl of ice cream. I'm sure, Jill, that you would want to have that too.

JILL: Well, sure.

THERAPIST: Or maybe not.

JILL: Yeah, I like ice cream.

THERAPIST: So I think that those are opportunities, when you guys are present, for her to have these kinds of food, so then, if she's feeling like the eating disorder, the little guy, wants her to get rid of what she just ate, you guys can be there and say, "Hey, what can we do to help you get over this urge?"

FATHER: Well, how do you talk to her about this? After she does eat a little of it, her tendency is to go upstairs.

THERAPIST: Let's talk about this.

JILL: I haven't gone up lately. I mean, most of the time I'm in my room because I just have to clean it all the time.

THERAPIST: But there could be an opportunity to get rid of it.

JILL: I guess there could. I mean, you could hear the toilet flush, but usually I'm cleaning my room because you can't even see the floor.

MOTHER: Or taking a nap.

JILL: Yeah, or taking a nap.

The parents have been quite successful at separating the illness from their daughter and also demonstrating a noncritical attitude toward her. For instance, Dad referred to the eating disorder symptoms as "the guy that comes out" or "That little guy, you said he's still going to be there, but maybe he's smaller than I thought," whereas Mother would talk about "it" when she referred to the bulimia. The degree to which this noncritical stance is due to their relationship prior to the onset of the illness, and/or the therapist succeeding in helping the parents understand this illness from the start of treatment, would be difficult to determine. Notwithstanding, with the therapist's modeling a noncritical stance throughout, both parents have been able to curtail their daughter's eating disorder by being quite "strict" with the bulimia without sacrificing their good relationship with their daughter. A good example of how the parents would combine humor with rules around curtailing the eating disorder is this dialogue from Dad: "Well, we could play tricks before we went to bed. If we were going to go to bed and she was going to be out late, we could move the cookies and put a little note. There's nothing wrong with her coming in late at night and having something healthy before she goes to bed."

Continue to Modify Parental and Sibling Criticisms

THERAPIST: But sometimes the eating disorder—and I'm not saying that this is what is happening with you, Jill—I know of young women who throw up in their rooms, finding a bag and getting rid of it in that way. It's just a very sneaky illness, and I know that sounds disgusting and you [the parents] think she would never do that, and Jill, you'd think, "I'd never do that," but sometimes it can be really strong. Even if you've had a period of time when that little guy has gone on vacation, it comes back to work because it can be that strong. So let's think of those times, like after she's eaten, what is it that you guys can do to help? It may be that you can't really rely on Jill to suggest "Let's go take a walk," because she may be conflicted, listening to the little guy or listening to the healthy part of her. What can you guys think about doing? I want you guys to feel like you're helping her to eat these foods, in moderation, and realize that she may feel guilty about that.

FATHER: It's just hard for us to be there, and if you're talking about at night, it's rare that all three of us will be sitting down at 8 o'clock at night. When are we there together? What are the odds that all three of us will be there for dinner? And then, after dinner, either plan something or talk, just so we know, hey, we just got done, maybe bring up the little guy, bring up purging, bring up whatever, just to talk about it so we know that. (*turning to Jill*) I think if you reminded yourself of it, or if we remind you of it, then you'd have the tendency of not wanting to do it because we just got finished talking about it.

MOTHER: I think we have been doing that—just our presence at a critical time, like right after dinner, has made a big impact. I'm usually home and, like I was saying in the beginning, I felt like I had to get her away from home, for example, go shopping or play scrabble, and we did do that. So for a couple of weeks we did some intense things to keep her busy. But now we've gone back just to our presence and just us being there.

THERAPIST: Is it helpful?

MOTHER: Yes, it has been helpful and we do talk, because in the beginning we wouldn't talk about it. Not that we talk about it a lot, but we're comfortable talking about it. And we're comfortable saying to her, "How are you doing?" And she'll say "Fine," and I suppose when I say, "How are you doing?" it is the way I say it. I don't have to say, "How's the eating disorder?" She knows it's different from "How are you today?" She knows what we mean when we say, "How are you doing?"

THERAPIST: So it's a special tone, meaning "How is the guy?"

MOTHER: Yes, and "Are you doing okay?" and "Are you filling out your log?" Both of us are doing a lot of that, and we can see too that she's doing a good job, and handling it, and she's come a long way.

The above passages are a very good example of two noncritical parents who are full of praise for their daughter and her efforts to overcome her bulimia. They have been successful at separating the illness from their daughter and have made some practical changes in their day-to-day routines to make sure that they are available, both physically and emotionally, to help Jill overcome her eating disorder. Their positive tone continues in the ensuing passages.

Continue to Distinguish the Patient and Her Interests from Those of BN

THERAPIST: She certainly has. I know that a lot of this treatment has focused on what your parents do to help you with your eating disorder. But I also want to recognize the reasons why we see zeros [in reference to the binge/purge log] is because you really want to get better from this too. You're really trying not to binge and purge as well. I don't want to say that we're out of the woods yet, and I think that's why we want to think about, particularly with summer coming, where it's going to be more unstructured, how we can help make sure that the progress you've made thus far continues. So we're going on this upward trajectory, as opposed to going down.

FATHER: I think it's going to be more dangerous in the summer because, in the winter, the way I look at this, when you wear a lot of clothes, a lot of sweaters, a lot of pants, you don't really look at yourself as much. In the summer it's hot and all you have on is shorts and short tops, so you look at yourself a lot more. If you don't like what you see, you'll tend to freak out. Is that going to bring the bingeing on? I think it's more critical in the summertime.

THERAPIST: That's a very good point.

MOTHER: That and the unstructuredness, if that's a word.

THERAPIST: Yes, the two things.

MOTHER: The summer is very unstructured. She'll stay out, I know she will. She's 18 now, and it's hard for us to just let go.

THERAPIST: I think, Jill, it's very helpful for you to know that this is a temporary treatment. We realize that you are 18 and this seems very unorthodox to be giving your parents control over this portion of your life, monitoring your food or where you are going after you eat. But I also think there can be a balance of respecting your wanting to go out with your friends in the evening, for instance. This is provided that you guys know that she's had a good dinner and have monitored her for an hour or so after she's eaten and know that it stayed down. She didn't binge, she didn't purge, so okay, she can go out with her friends. It can be a kind of reward for her, because I don't want you to feel that any of this is punishment for being sick; you're continually having to watch television with your parents or play Scrabble with them every single summer night—though, I know you guys have a good relationship.

MOTHER: I think that's a good point, and I'm glad you're saying that. Actually, I'm thinking, again about summer. Since the kids were little, and being a teacher, I remember September coming and thinking, "I'm glad summer's over because we need structure again." Our summers are typically very unstructured, and I see what you're saying now. We need to keep our meals somewhat more structured.

THERAPIST: I think it's good practice for you to be helping Jill so that she'll learn, herself, when she's at college, where it's a much more unstructured environment than high school. You guys can rest assured that she's going to be in Massachusetts and she's going to be eating meals and snacks, not restricting eating during the day and then having the eating disorder and having to binge and purge. She doesn't want that, for sure, and you guys don't want that.

MOTHER: I think the other good thing is that we have a good enough rapport with Jill that when she does go to college, we're still going to talk about this, even if it is just on the phone. Both of us are going to say, "Well, how are you doing?" And she's going to know what we mean. And I trust her that she will be honest with us.

THERAPIST: Provided that the eating disorder has receded somewhat.

MOTHER: Well, that's true.

In the preceding passages, the therapist did a good job of praising the patient and the parents for their efforts at combating the eating disorder. However, she does caution the family that they are not "out of the woods just yet." The therapist is helping the family plan for the more unstructured time ahead of them (summer) and helped them to brainstorm how to help Jill during these times. It is also a good way to move the discussion to the issue of Jill leaving home and going off to college in the fall (the therapist jumps this far ahead just briefly) and, in so doing, helps the family plan for the summer and to use that as a springboard for Jill's eventual departure for college in the fall. Introducing these topics is also moving the treatment closer to the end of Phase I; the therapist is bringing up topics that are more typically discussed in Phases II and III. In these passages the therapist also demonstrates great respect for the adolescent and reminds her that Phase I interventions are temporary.

Discuss and Support Parents' Efforts at Reestablishing Healthy Eating

THERAPIST: Let's think about dinners. Do you guys have a plan for after dinner, because that's the danger area. Once she's eaten something nutritious, maybe that would be a good opportunity for you to have her eat one of the foods that it's hard to eat on her own, even though she has done it, like ice cream or cookies. That sounds like a danger area after she's had dinner. Can you all put your collective heads together and think of ways to make this work? Jill, you have a say in this too. We want this to be a collaborative.

FATHER: Well, one way to do it is to say that the end of dinner would be an hour later. So, if we're done eating at 7:15, we could say, "Okay, wait, we're not going anywhere, we still have to talk about whatever." Or maybe what we'll do is, when we're done eating, we have to spend the next half hour doing something together; "What do you want to do this time? Want to go for a walk or sit here and do dishes and talk?"

We have to guarantee that we'll spend the next 45 minutes, from the time the last person is done eating, together, if it's doing something, just walking in the neighborhood, doing dishes, playing Scrabble, whatever, doing something. The end of the meal is going to be when we're done with that. Then we're done.

MOTHER: Since that hour, or 45 minutes, is the most critical time, you're saying to keep her busy or within our sight?

THERAPIST: Yes, and also, so that you guys have the reassurance of knowing, "That was a good dinner she ate and she kept it down." We want to make sure that she keeps it down, that this little guy doesn't have any opportunity. It may be present, but you're going to say you're not welcome here at the table.

FATHER: I think, even if you had dinner, then something that would help you move would be good.

THERAPIST: Like a walk or something like that?

FATHER: Yes.

THERAPIST: That certainly could be an option. What do you think, Mrs. Kenny? Jill, I also want to get your view of what your dad must said.

MOTHER: I suppose part of me is thinking that (*turning to Jill*), and I could ask you this, when you did the purging, was it dinner?

JILL: No, well sometimes, but no.

THERAPIST: It wasn't usually purging?

JILL: If I had a lot of cookies after dinner, but not if I had, like, a turkey sandwich.

MOTHER: It wasn't usually purging dinner, it was usually purging something sweet?

JILL: If I ate food afterward, I usually would purge, but I don't do it anymore.

MOTHER: It was usually the after-dinner food.

THERAPIST: Sure.

MOTHER: So, if dinner was over at 7, it was more at 7:30 that she started. She would have a bowl of ice cream or some cookies. I remember it, five times into the kitchen to get something. We talked about her binges not being huge amounts, but to her they were, so that's what it was. So maybe at 9 o'clock she was doing that or 10 o'clock, or even later. But I heard what you said earlier, that we need to establish regular eating patterns, because if you don't eat all day, you're going to be too hungry. We always knew that part of this was establishing better eating habits and nutrition.

THERAPIST: Also, integrating some of these ice cream and cookies so that they're not so forbidden or you deprive yourself of them so much that, when you're given an opportunity, you feel, "I can't eat just one cookie, I have to eat 10." If you have a dessert at dinner, and you're with her, and the eating disorder makes her feel like "If I'd just had the dinner, I'd be fine, but the dessert pushed me over," then you guys can be with her. If she's feeling that way, there's not going to be an opportunity for her to get rid of it. She'll also have experience with eating those things in moderation and being okay with it. Jill, what do you feel? I want to talk to your parents, but I also want to get your read. Your dad thinks there can be choices of what you can do afterward.

JILL: Yes, that's fine. Usually, I don't know; on the weekends I'll eat there and then go get ready to go out. I don't really want to hang out there until 9 o'clock and then say, "All right I'm going to get ready now."

THERAPIST: But would that be something you're willing to do to make sure?

JILL: I'm not going to purge. Really, I don't want to hang out until 9 o'clock and not go out, and then start getting ready. Do you really think it's that big of a deal that we need to make sure that I keep my spaghetti in my stomach? I don't know, I easily can eat dinner and go get ready, shower.

MOTHER: I think I learned that what is important is making sure we're eating normally.

JILL: Normal meals?

MOTHER: Yes, normal meals at normal times.

JILL: We have done a lot of that.

MOTHER: I think that that is important. And, you know, we're a pretty close family and we do things together, even, I think unconsciously, that first hour after dinner.

JILL: Yes, we usually do something.

MOTHER: We usually do the dishes or, especially with it being nice out now, everyone's kind of doing their own thing. You [Dad] might be washing the car, I might be watering my flowers, and she [Jill] might be just watching TV.

THERAPIST: So it sounds like you're already a close family, and this won't be a shocker. Because sometimes with families it becomes like this: "No way are we spending time together!"

JILL: Yeah, we don't have to have it be like "Okay, now I have to go hang out with my mom and dad."

THERAPIST: I'm glad you brought that up.

JILL: It's just normal. We don't have to worry about it, then.

MOTHER: And I want her to have choices.

THERAPIST: Absolutely.

MOTHER: Because there have been choices when I've said to her, "Do you want to go for a walk?" I want to walk. I try to exercise. A couple of times she said "No," and I don't want to force her, but a couple of times she said, "Yeah." Even last Saturday we went.

JILL: Rollerblading, well, I went rollerblading.

MOTHER: We went to Wicker Park and then Sunday, we went to the Forest Reserve. So I have to accept if sometimes she doesn't want to do an activity with me. That's what happened with the scrapbook too.

JILL: Sometimes I'm in the mood, and then sometimes I'm not.

MOTHER: (*repeating*) Sometimes she's in the mood, and sometimes she's not!

THERAPIST: Could there be a compromise? Sometimes it really isn't appealing to go for a walk with your mom or do something with your dad. You could do something on your own, but your mom and dad would know that the eating disorder wasn't going to get you to go upstairs and get rid of the food? I know we're talking to a healthy Jill right now, so it seems absurd, like, "I'm not going to get rid of my spaghetti, so why are we having this discussion?" But it's really sneaky. It comes up and just bites you on the butt, and I think we just all really need to problem-solve for this. It doesn't have to be some chart you've made up, like, *"Okay, tonight we're going to play Scrabble or learn a language,"* but I think it is important for there to be some structure so that you guys are sure that the eating disorder doesn't sneak its way in and make her get rid of something.

MOTHER: I think the other thing that's happening is that—and maybe this is why we're feeling this way—I think all of us are able to recognize this little guy.

JILL: Yeah.

In the preceding passages the therapist carefully helps the parents and the adolescent to work out a way in which they (the parents) can spend time with Jill after mealtimes to prevent purging. Everyone is very careful to figure out a way to do this that would not be experienced by Jill as punitive. The therapist makes sure to solicit Jill's response to her parents' suggestions. Although she protests at first, this does not last very long, and the good nature of this family allows all of them to conclude that they are a "pretty close family and we do things together." The emphasis in this part of the session is on the pragmatics of helping the family think about regular meals and how to incorporate forbidden foods as they attempt to help Jill overcome the illness.

Close All Sessions by Recounting of Progress

THERAPIST: That's great progress.

MOTHER: [referring to Jill's progress] I think she's doing it, and I think he and I are doing it too. We can start to see it. It's always there, so we're very conscious of it. When I really needed to say to her, "I want you to be with me for an hour right now," it's because I recognize that the little guy was sitting on her shoulder.

JILL: Right.

THERAPIST: I think that's really very true. You have a close relationship. I think that you can sense when it's hard for Jill in some instances, but I also think that, in this stage that we're in here, if you give the illness an opportunity, it's going to take it. I want you, Jill, to be able to go off to college and not have any symptoms, so you don't have to worry about it. You're taking care of it now; your mom and dad have said this: We really want to take care of this now so it's not an issue. It's still going to be there, but we've really done some good work together.

MOTHER: I think that we're sensing that we have done good work. I think it's good, and I think we all know it's important that we come every week to listen and talk about it just because of what you're saying. We all understand that it can come back. Maybe we're getting a little too complacent.

THERAPIST: Well, I think you guys have made remarkable progress. I think, even before treatment started, you really worked hard on this. However, I think there is a tendency to get complacent, feeling like everything's out of the way, but it's still in the room.

MOTHER: Which is why treatment is still necessary as we go through the next couple of months.

THERAPIST: Right, exactly. And there are phases of this process, absolutely, so that your parents spend less time monitoring what you're doing or spending time with you engaged in activities for the purpose of diverting the little guy. I think right now it's important to not give the eating disorder any room to breathe. And I'm glad you raised the issue of summer coming up because I think . . .

MOTHER: Because that will be a lot of change.

THERAPIST: You're right, a lot of change.

MOTHER: I think it will be very interesting the next couple of weeks, because she basically only has, what, 2 days left? She has finals next week, then she graduates next Friday.

THERAPIST: Okay, well, this week let's think about your continuing efforts to work together, trying to do that, and then we can talk about what we can do about the lunch when summer comes. Like I said, this is very collaborative here, and Jill, this is not supposed to be this prison sentence either, because it's summer and it's your last summer before college. That's important, but I also want to recognize the importance of getting this thing under control.

MOTHER: I think, of all of us, she's feeling that she's cured. Right?

THERAPIST: That's wonderful, that's great.

MOTHER: I think we're supportive of that too, but I think he and I are a little bit more . . . and you also, the three of us are more reluctant to say she's 100% cured. But I think she thinks she is cured.

THERAPIST: And that's great. I think that's so wonderful, we just need to make sure that progress continues. Let's just fortify our efforts here and get this taken care of so there's no chance of this illness coming back. One of my families says, "We just want to strangle it, to make sure it never comes back, never has air any more." So that's it, thanks so much for being here, and I look forward to seeing you in 2 weeks.

The therapist ends this session on a positive note because the patient is making good progress, and everybody is recognizing the improvement. The therapist expresses some caution, though, that the eating disorder is not entirely out of the way, a sentiment that is echoed by the parents. In this session, which is very typical of the first phase of treatment, the patient shows good progress and the therapist has begun to move things forward a little as she addressed the more unstructured summer coming up, as well as the patient leaving for college in the fall. If progress continues at this trend, this family would probably spend just a few more sessions in Phase I, with everyone agreeing that progress is on track, before moving to Phase II, in which they will all work together to hand over control eating back to Jill and to phase out the post meal supervision. These issues, among others, are the topic of the next few chapters.

CHAPTER 10

Phase II

Helping the Adolescent Eat on Her Own
(Sessions 11–16)

The patient's agreement to work with her parents to adhere to a balanced food intake, the absence of binge eating and purging, and familial relief that progress is being made all signal the start of the second phase of treatment. As was the case in Phase I of treatment, the therapist advises the parents that the main task in Phase II of treatment is to continue to work toward improving the health of their child. The focus of treatment during this phase remains firmly on eating disorder symptoms, albeit now in a family context that is characterized with decreased tension and stress. At the same time the therapist can now bring forward more general issues of adolescence, insofar as they directly relate to eating disorder symptoms (e.g., puberty, peer relations, and sexuality). Although directly addressing adolescent issues is the main aim of Phase III, the therapist should begin to make a transition to these matters toward the end of Phase II.

In order to reinforce the adolescent's developing autonomy and the family's success in Phase I, increased independence from the therapist is warranted. Therefore, sessions during Phase II should generally be scheduled 2–3 weeks apart. The therapist continues to weigh the patient at the start of every other session and to collect a report of binge eating and purging at each session. However, the need for therapeutic assistance is variable, and the therapist may find that intervals between sessions range from 1 to 6 weeks during this phase.

The attitude of the therapist in Phase II differs from the highly serious one displayed during most of Phase I. Because the patient and her family are succeeding in establishing healthy eating and curtailing bulimic behavior, the therapist is more optimistic and hopeful. From a developmental perspective, BN can be seen as having disrupted usual adolescent processes (i.e., increased independence, heightened importance of peer relations, and personal academic or vocational goals). In Phase II, the therapist begins to integrate the focus on eating disorder symptoms with pertinent events occurring in the adolescent's life as she begins to have an increased opportunity for independence and peer relationships—that is, problems of eating without restriction, binge eating or purging at school, when attending dances, or on dates. The specific issues the therapist is likely to address depend on the age and maturity of the adolescent as well as how quickly parental monitoring can be withdrawn safely; however, general guidelines about therapeutic procedures the therapist may employ are described below.

Often the patient's attitude has toward the therapist changes near the outset of Phase II. Whereas the patient was more guarded, even at times hostile, toward the therapist at the beginning of treatment, by Phase II her attitude is usually friendlier and more accepting. If the parents believe the therapist has helped them in their struggle with BN, this added confidence might help to spur them on as the move beyond the immediate problems that bulimia has caused them and turn to helping their adolescent begin to negotiate food-related issues in the context of their adolescent activities. Toward the end of the Phase II, the patient will have taken charge of her own eating and weight-related behaviors at an age-appropriate level, and the therapist should step back to allow the parents and adolescent to assume a more central role in treatment. In this way, the therapist and family can identify and amplify the adolescent's strengths and skills during the remaining sessions. In some cases the patient and family are now ready to take up the challenges of adolescence that the advent of BN interrupted. Once again aligned with her peers, and less preoccupied with the thoughts and behaviors of BN, the patient can begin to grapple with puberty, peer relationships, psychological autonomy, sexuality, and other typical issues of adolescence. At this point the parents may feel able to take a step back and watch their daughter address these issues with greater independence from them.

How Does the Therapist Assess the Family's Readiness for Phase II?

The following criteria are general guidelines that usually signal readiness for beginning Phase II:

- The patient is able, to a significant degree, to abstain from binge eating and purging (i.e., binges/purges less than one or two times a month).
- Weight is stable within broadly acceptable norms.
- The patient eats at regular intervals without excessive need for parental involvement, and the parents report no significant struggles to get the patient to eat regular meals.
- The parents report that they feel able to help the patient manage her bulimic behaviors; that is, the parents demonstrate a sense of relief that they can manage this illness.

How Does the Treatment Team Change in Phase II?

The treatment team for Phase II (the family therapy team plus the consulting team) remains intact. In this phase the physician is likely seeing the patient less frequently because immediate concerns about medical problems have decreased at this point. Typically, the physician might see the patient every 3–4 weeks at this point and let the therapist know if new medical problems are developing. The therapist, in turn, would report on behavioral progress and let the physician know if symptoms appeared to be worsening at any point. Patients who are taking medications are usually on a stable dose by this point and, as with the physician, meetings with the child psychiatrist typically occur less frequently. Contact between the therapist and child psychiatrist should continue at reasonable intervals, depending on the degree of concern, to ensure that the maximal benefit of medications and therapy is obtained. As the eating disorder dissipates, treatment begins to resemble usual family therapy for adolescents, and the involvement of the consulting team (e.g., the pediatrician or the nutritionist) may become more secondary. However, the reappearance of BN symptoms might necessitate reactivating the consulting team on a more regular basis. Therefore, all team members should be kept abreast of the patient's progress. The relationship among family therapy team members, though, remains essentially unchanged from Phase I to Phase II.

The major goals of Phase II of treatment are:

- To maintain parental management of eating disorder symptoms until patient shows evidence that she is able to eat in healthy ways and to do independently.
- To return control of food and weight to the adolescent.
- To explore relationship between adolescent developmental issues and BN.

In order to achieve these goals, the therapist undertakes the following interventions:

1. Weigh patient at the beginning of each session and collect binge/purge log.
2. Continue to support and assist parents in management of eating disorder symptoms until adolescent is able to eat well on her own without binge eating or purging.
3. Assist parents and adolescent in negotiating the return of control over eating to the adolescent.
4. Encourage family members to examine relationships between adolescent issues and the development of BN in their adolescent.
5. Continue to modify parental and sibling criticism of patient, especially in relation to the task of returning control of eating to patient.
6. Continue to assist siblings in supporting their ill sibling.
7. Continue to highlight difference between adolescent's own ideas and needs and those associated with BN.
8. Close sessions with positive support.

Although the treatment goals are the same for all needed sessions of this phase, the emphasis of each session changes as the family moves toward the end of this phase. For example, sessions may start out very similar to those of Phase I, with a review of eating habits and bulimic symptoms as the primary goal, but the emphasis will shift toward self-maintenance of regular and healthy eating as control over this area is handed back to the patient.

Finally, the therapist will begin to focus more on adolescent issues as she/he makes a transfer from Phase II to Phase III.

Weigh the Patient at the Beginning of Every Session and Collect Binge/Purge Log

Why

As in the previous phase, continued close monitoring of binge eating and purging (every session) using the patient's binge/purge log, and weight (every other session), is an important mechanism for providing feedback to the patient and family on progress.

How

At this point, the patient and therapist should have developed an increased rapport such that checking on binge eating and purging becomes increasingly acceptable. The intimacy of sharing this vulnerable information should also lead to greater trust overall. As this phase begins, the adolescent is often more interested in discussing her wishes to be rewarded for her compliance with parental demands for healthy eating by gaining increasing control over this process once again. The therapist should be receptive to these wishes without committing to a course of action in response to them, other than assuring the patient that the parental control of food and weight will eventually end. The therapist's binge/purge charts document progress toward this end and therefore provides an opportunity to help generate a realistic perspective on the achievements of the family to date. On the other hand, the therapist can assume that not everything that is happening in treatment is related to binge/purge and weight stabilization of the patient, especially during this phase of treatment. Therefore, as this phase continues, emphasis on these checks may also decrease.

Continue to Support and Assist Parents in Management of Eating Disorder Symptoms until Adolescent Is Able to Eat Well on Her Own without Binge Eating and Purging

Why

Maintaining healthy eating and abstaining from bulimic symptoms remain fragile at the early stage of Phase II, because complete abstinence from binge eating and purging has not usually been achieved. Therefore, the therapist has to make sure that the parents do not relax their efforts to reestablish healthy eating habits and extinguish binge eating and purging. Although this task is very similar to that described in Phase I, the therapist should note the shift in emphasis here. Whereas in Phase I the therapist's task was that of directly helping and coaching the parents to get their daughter to eat in healthy ways, the therapist's role here shifts more toward that of greater delegation. That is, the therapist steps back somewhat from taking an active a role in facilitating parental management of eating disorders; instead, the therapist aims to enhance and consolidate the parents' trust in their own abilities to make appropriate decisions in the process of reestablishing healthy eating in their daughter. This shift is particularly important because the next therapeutic task is to support the parents as they negotiate with their daughter about how to return control over eating back to her.

How

The therapist starts this phase of treatment with the same goal in mind as in Phase I: to systematically review and reinforce the parents' efforts at reestablishing healthy eating in their daughter. The therapist insists that the parents remain consistent in their efforts to restore the consumption of three balanced meals, until he/she is convinced that the patient no longer doubts the parents' ability and resolve to prevent her from engaging in abnormal eating patterns that precipitate bulimic behaviors. The therapist remains focused on the BN symptoms for now. Sessions consist of a careful and thorough review of events surrounding eating. These reviews are now aimed at examining the procedures being used by the parents to help their daughter begin to take control of eating more independently. The family's strategies to bring about this recovery process should dominate discussions for as long as it is appropriate. For instance, each family member should be asked about events of the past week and how she/he has gone about the task of reestablishing healthy eating. In the same style of *circular questioning*, as outlined before, each response should be verified with every family member to determine how he or she would describe events. Discrepancies should be carefully examined because their clarifications are helpful for the therapist in selecting and reinforcing those steps the parents will have to take to improve their efforts. As before, the therapist should use these sessions to carefully bolster the parents in their knowledge of nutritious and balanced meals and reinforce their efforts to bring about healthy eating and decreases in binge eating and purging.

It is also important to involve the adolescent in this process by taking into account "what's in it" for her. The therapist helps the family to identify ways to motivate cooperation by promoting the adolescent's reentry into age-appropriate activities, particularly with peers. For example, parents now encourage their daughter to attend parties and dances and go on dates. During this phase, questions about when it is appropriate for the patient to resume exercise and at what level of frequency and intensity often arise. Although there are no definitive rules about how to approach this issue in BN, a general guideline would recommend eating sufficient amounts to have enough energy to exercise and avoiding the possibility that exercise becomes a way of purging. Applying this guideline usually means that the adolescent exercises no more than 30 minutes several times a week. If the adolescent is on a competitive sports team, gradually increasing the frequency and duration of exercise on a weekly basis is generally a safe way to proceed. Because osteopenia and osteoporosis occur in BN (Zipfel, Lowe, & Herzog, 2005) (though exact rates for these problems are not yet known), caution about possible injury during exercise needs to be stressed as the parents relinquish their supervision over these activities.

Assist Parents and Adolescent in Negotiating the Return of Control over Eating to the Adolescent

Why

The task of reestablishing healthy eating (as described in Phase I) is continued during Phase II, although with a gradual change in emphasis. Soon in Phase II, the therapist will guide the family toward *relinquishing* its control over the patient's eating. This shift can only be initiated if the patient's weight is stable, eating habits are healthy, bulimic symptoms are largely under control, and the therapist is assured that improvement will continue even when the parents begin to exert less vigilance. Once the patient is relatively free from the behaviors associated with BN, parents are encouraged to allow the patient to function with increasing independence in relation to her level of adolescent development. For example, the parents of a patient in high school might allow her to have lunch off campus with her friends, whereas during Phase I they required her to come home for lunch during the school day. Also, the gradual phasing out of parental supervision should serve as a trial period to see whether the adolescent copes well with eating adequately on her own, without the reappearance of eating disorder symptomatology that thwarts her progress.

The therapist's aim is to assist the parents and the adolescent to bring about a careful and mutually agreed upon handing over of responsibility for eating-related activities from the parents to the adolescent. This process is orchestrated against the backdrop of each family's unique rituals or habits around regular eating activities (before the eating disorder changed the family's mealtimes) and the age of the adolescent as well as the degree of recovery he/she has experienced. Although the parents seek guidance from the therapist about how to proceed with handing control of eating back to the patient, it is ultimately the parents *in collaboration* with the patient who should decide how to proceed with this process. This is a delicate maneuver as the therapist balances the involvement of the patient, who might jump at the opportunity to regain responsibility in food choices, the parents, and her/himself in terms of the decision-making process.

How

Parents may choose to gradually lesson their control over this process in several ways, for example, by letting the patient dish up for herself at mealtimes while the parents continue to supervise this activity. Alternatively, parents can allow the adolescent more control over food choices as long as the selections represent healthy and adequate quantities of food. Another way to move forward is for the parents to leave the patient to her own devices when it comes to one or two meals per day, while still supervising the main meal of the day. The parents will have suspended their supervision after mealtimes or in terms of bathroom visits at this point in the recovery process. Ultimately, the parents and the patient would want to arrive at age-appropriate decisions that are in keeping with each family's unique set of rules about food shopping, food preparation, joint family meals versus individual responsibility and tastes, and so on.

Encourage Family Members to Examine Relationships between Adolescent Issues and the Development of BN in Their Adolescent

Why

Once eating ceases to be the sole focus of discussions, the therapist helps the family to negotiate important adolescent issues that have been deferred until now, but only in the limited context of those that relate directly to eating and weight control (e.g., eating at school, shopping for dresses for a formal dance). Overall, the patient is encouraged to engage in age-appropriate socialization as much as possible and as soon as possible. Depending on the age of onset, the BN symptoms have usually interfered with some aspect of the patient's normal psychosocial and psychosexual development. For instance, adolescents with BN usually have distorted concerns about their bodies and their sexual attractiveness, leading them to sometimes to avoid dating or any activities that involve skimpy clothing (e.g., going to a swimming pool). During Phase II the focus is more directly on understanding the relationship of the symptoms of BN and the dilemmas of adolescent life (e.g., dating, parties, prom dresses) in order to diminish the salience of these normal adolescent events in maintaining BN.

How

One example in which these issues can begin to be explored, within the context of a continuing focus on the eating disorder, is adolescent dating. Although dating in itself is representative of many important issues in adolescent development (e.g., individuation and psychosexual maturation), the patient can only successfully embark on this course when the eating is no longer of concern. At this point in treatment, the therapist will not discuss the more general issues about adolescent behaviors but rather concentrate on whether all concerned are reassured that going out for dinner with a partner can be done knowing that the patient will make appropriate food choices. The therapist should let the parents and patient problem-solve in session to work out a plan in terms of the choice of restaurant and the food items that will be ordered while she is out on a date. In addition, the patient should have a plan worked out beforehand as to how she will prevent herself from either bingeing or purging. This way, parental anxiety will be diminished and the patient will experience a decreased need to eat less on a date as a way of showing others that she can control her eating and weight and instead remain focused on nurturing her fragile recovery from her eating disorder.

Continue to Modify Parental and Sibling Criticism of Patient, Especially in Relation to the Task of Returning Control of Eating to Patient

Why

The general reason that family criticism is suspected to contribute to poorer outcome was discussed in Chapter 4. In the context of Phase II, how the therapist manages any family criticism is determined by comments made about the adolescent as she resumes eating on her own. As the patient begins to regain control and autonomy over her eating, there is renewed opportunity for parents and siblings to reproach her and thereby compromise her best efforts. Critical responses may undermine the patient's attempts to return to healthy eating, exacerbate the bulimic symptoms, and trigger greater resistance to accepting help from her family. Sometimes as the adolescent becomes more independent, he/she expresses more defiance of parental authority, which in turn can trigger parental criticism; hence, the therapist needs to keep the focus on minimizing parental and sibling criticism in Phase II.

How

The basic mechanisms for modifying parental and sibling criticism have been described above. During this phase, especially as the adolescent is encouraged to resume eating on her own, the therapist can model approval and acceptance of her struggle by saying, for example:

"You made a great effort to gain control over your binge eating. Now we just have to focus on the few remaining issues that make complete abstinence difficult for you."

Or, alternatively:

"It seems your parents have high expectations of you, and although part of you wishes to meet them, in other ways you may feel that you can never achieve them. This may frustrate you and them at times and lead to conflicts, although your goals are the same—that is, to help you get your life as a teenager back."

On the other hand, if the therapist needs to address the adolescent about being unreasonably oppositional, she/he might ask:

"It has been hard to have your parents so involved in your eating, hasn't it? Do you think sometimes you are fighting with them now because you resented that?"

Continue to Assist Siblings in Supporting Their Ill Sibling

Why

The previous chapters detailed the siblings' key role in therapy and why they should support their ill sibling. However, as the bulimic adolescent clearly improves, the siblings may feel that their work is done. It is true that the need for their specific support in relation to helping the adolescent with tolerating her parents' control over eating-related behavior diminishes in Phase II. Nonetheless, the adolescent has not yet recovered and still needs support, especially when she advocates for more autonomy. Siblings are still important in helping her to sustain her progress during this process.

How

The strategies for involving siblings have been illustrated earlier. At this point, it is usually only necessary to continue to bring up the issue for brief discussion during every session. The therapist may inquire of each of the siblings, "What did you do that helped your sister feel better this week about herself?" It is helpful to explore in some detail both the thought behind the sibling's action as well as the ill adolescent's appreciation of, or lack thereof, the effort. If the patient has older brothers or sisters in the therapy, they are particularly useful in this phase because they often identify with the patient's more typical struggles of adolescence (now that BN is not at the center of it) and can support her needs for greater independence and empathize with her teenage dilemmas.

Continue to Highlight Difference between the Adolescent's Own Ideas and Needs and Those Associated with BN

Why

It continues to be important to highlight differences between bulimic-related thinking (extreme overvaluation of weight and shape and food) and the adolescent's own beliefs to clarify the parents' and adolescent's shared goals for growth and development. However, during this phase, it is usually much clearer to the family and patient where bulimic thinking diverges from typical adolescent concerns about independence and social relations with peers. The rationale for continuing to separate bulimic thinking and usual adolescent concerns is, as before, to decrease adolescent shame about having developed BN and encouraging the family to see the problem as BN and not the adolescent herself.

How

The therapist emphasizes the differences between BN-related thinking and goals and those of the adolescent by facilitating a negotiation between the adolescent and the parents that allows the adolescent to safely regain control of eating-related activities from parents. Thus, the therapist encourages the adolescent to set her own goals for recovery; for example, regaining the privilege to attend a school camp that BN deprived her of because of her severe malnutrition. In addition, the therapist should explore failure to achieve such goals as a way to invigorate the adolescent's own wish to differentiate herself from BN.

Close Sessions with Positive Support

Why

As in previous sessions, the attitude of the therapists at the conclusion of sessions is warm and generally congratulatory so that guilt, powerlessness, and feelings of inadequacy are minimized. By being positive and encouraging, the therapist also helps to ensure that family members continue to feel valued, which helps keep them committed to coming to therapy, despite being exhausted or tempted to turn to other pressing problems.

How

As in previous sessions, the therapist summarizes the main achievements of the family while footnoting the shortcomings. This is done efficiently, but with warmth, as the family gets ready to depart. The therapist may say something like the following:

> "You have done wonderful work today in figuring out how to help your daughter get prepared to return to school next week. You have also made it clear that you have been challenged at times by her demands for immediate and complete autonomy. As you struggle with this issue over the next 2 weeks, keep in mind that the struggle is against the illness of bulimia and not with one another."

The therapist takes care to say goodbye to each family member as she/he leaves the room in order that each continues to feel recognized and valued.

End-of-Session Review

As was the case for all sessions in the first phase of treatment, the lead therapist should continue to review treatment progress at regular intervals with other members of the team to make sure that everyone agrees that progress is occurring as expected and that any new problems are identified.

Common Questions and Troubleshooting for Phase II

• *What if the patient shows renewed resistance to parents' efforts?* Some patients, due to prior experience of feeling decreased stress and anxiety post bingeing or post vomiting, may resist any further efforts by their parents to bring these behaviors under control and reestablish healthy eating habits. The therapist should use this opportunity to illustrate the severity of the problems that BN is creating to emphasize the need for parents to stay the course of controlling these behaviors. Therapists may remind parents, for example, of the medical complications of persistent vomiting, such as low potassium, dehydration, loss of teeth, and esophageal tears. The purpose of this intervention is to once again raise their anxiety and reinvigorate them in their efforts to bring about healthy eating in their adolescent offspring.

- *What if the patient regains independence in eating and then starts anew with a cycle of dieting, binge eating, and purging?* Throughout this phase the parents and the patient should be prepared for a cyclical presentation of the BN, which is common, and told that the treatment will give them tools to help with future recurrences of the bulimic behaviors. Cyclical bulimic symptoms may be a poor prognostic sign. To reduce the likelihood of a cyclic pattern, it is imperative that independence in eating not be prematurely returned to the patient. Although the choice of how the parents relinquish control to the patient should ideally be worked out between the parents and patient, the therapist should provide consultation about the timing as well as the tempo of this process. However, should the patient return to a dieting, binge eating, and purging cycle after control over eating has been returned to her, it would demonstrate to everyone that this step was premature. The therapist should reinvigorate the parents swiftly and have them reestablish control over their daughter's eating. The therapist and the parents should strive *not* to appear punitive. After all, it is the therapist and parents who misjudged the patient's readiness to proceed without constant supervision of her eating. The therapist should note, however, that it is relatively uncommon for a return to starvation, binge eating, and purging to occur if the transition to independent eating has been negotiated mutually and carefully.

- *What if the parents start to depend too much on the therapist to solve problems?* Throughout treatment the therapist reinforces the parents' ability to arrive at their own solutions to restore their daughter's health. For most parents this strategy enhances parental self-efficacy and supports their independence. However, some parents may nonetheless defer to the therapist for consultation and advice at the expense of their own empowerment. In these cases, the therapist will use the few sessions in Phase II to help the parents problem-solve *in sessions* so that they have the opportunity to arrive at their own solutions.

- *What is the best way to focus and contain adolescent themes appropriately?* The therapist may be anxious to move treatment onto a different emphasis and introduce adolescent themes at a time when reestablishing healthy eating and refraining from binge eating and purging are still too tentative. Further, the patient may see a diversion of attention from BN as a potential opportunity to reinvigorate attempts at bulimic behaviors. This shift would be unfortunate because it would signal the therapist to once more return to interventions appropriate for the first goal of this phase— that is, consistent parental management of BN symptoms—and inevitably delay the treatment process. On the other hand, the therapist also has an opportunity in Phase III to deal with adolescent issues and not be distracted. The family and adolescent should be reassured that these themes/issues will be contained, managed, and better explored in Phase III.

• *How does the therapist maintain his/her focus, keep the whole family engaged, and make a graceful move toward Phase III?* This point can be a difficult part of treatment because all parties concerned (i.e., the family and the therapist) might be exhausted after months of maintaining a diligent focus on the BN symptoms. With the patient's BN under control, the therapist may have to ward off her/his own desire, as well as that of the family, to curtail any further treatment. However, as we have stated earlier on, we believe that BN has disrupted normal adolescent development to some degree, and an important part of successful treatment is to make sure that the patient is well on her way, with the help of her parents and her siblings, to negotiating adolescence once more. Whether this is a short and limited process or a more involved and elaborate one, the therapist aims to ensure the patient's successful return to adolescence (which is the central focus of Phase III).

Conclusion of Phase II

Most adolescent issues deferred to until now are explored more thoroughly in Phase III. The patient and the family's readiness to progress to Phase III is indicated when

1. The patient eats regular meals without parental supervision.
2. Bulimic symptoms are absent, and weight is maintained between 95 and 105% ideal body weight (IBW).
3. The family is able to discuss non-eating-related adolescent issues.
4. The patient shows a strong alliance with her peers.

When these indicators of progress are in place, the therapist will begin to transition the family work to focus on more general issues of adolescent development as they begin Phase III.

CHAPTER 11

Phase II in Action

This chapter provides an example of a session in Phase II. It begins with a brief review of the past week or so during which the therapist has an opportunity to meet with the adolescent on her own. At this stage of treatment, the patient's eating is well under control and there is more room for her and the therapist to talk about general events and concerns. The parents join the session after a period of about 10 minutes. This session is divided into separate parts, as are most sessions during this phase of the treatment, based on the specific intervention used. In addition, explanatory notes are added as the session unfolds to highlight the specific aims the therapist has in mind.

As a reminder, the three main goals for this session are:

- To maintain parental management of BN symptoms until patient shows evidence that she is able to eat in healthy ways and to do so independently.
- To return control of food and weight to the adolescent.
- To explore relationship between adolescent developmental issues and BN.

In order to achieve these goals, the therapist undertakes the following interventions:

1. Weigh patient at the beginning of each session and collect binge/purge log.
2. Continue to support and assist parents in management of eating

187

disorder symptoms until adolescent is able to eat well on her own without binge eating or purging.

3. Assist parents and adolescent in negotiating the return of control of eating-related behaviors to the adolescent.
4. Encourage family members to examine relationships between adolescent issues and the development of BN in their adolescent.
5. Continue to modify parental and sibling criticism of the patient, especially in relation to the task of returning control of eating to the patient.
6. Continue to assist siblings in supporting their ill sibling.
7. Continue to highlight difference between adolescent's own ideas and needs and those associated with BN.
8. Close sessions with positive support.

Note that even though the above interventions are all part of Phase II, it does not mean that the therapist will have an opportunity to implement each one in every session. For instance, in the case that follows, the patient's younger brother did not attend sessions in Phase II. Consequently, there was little, if any, opportunity to help the sibling continue to assist his sister during this phase of treatment. Also, Lisa's parents were not critical of her and left the therapist with few, if any, opportunities to ameliorate criticism. Therefore, the ensuing session provides the therapist with the opportunity to demonstrate most, but not all, of the typical Phase II interventions.

Clinical Background

Lisa is an 18-year-old Caucasian female presenting with a diagnosis of BN. Her height is 63 inches, and her weight is 138 pounds with a BMI of 24. Lisa states that ideally she would like to weigh 100 pounds. She lives with her parents and younger brother. Lisa presented to the clinic with bulimic symptoms that had begun 12 months ago, and she reports binge eating about once per day and self-induced vomiting about twice per day. Lisa does not report using laxatives, diuretics, or diet pills, but she did engage in compensatory exercise approximately once a week over the last month. In addition, Lisa was a frequent alcohol user in social settings, though she reported less drinking of late. A few months before treatment started, Lisa was smoking one and a half packs of cigarettes per day, but has since reduced smoking to one or two packs per month. She claimed to not be addicted. Lisa has regular periods and is not taking oral contraceptives. She denied any functional impairment as a result of her eating disorder and did not present with other comorbidities. However, she started treatment with Lexapro 20 mg, which was prescribed by a prior provider for "anxiety and mood" symptoms. Lisa and her family preferred to maintain this medication and dose level.

Weigh the Patient at the Beginning of Each Session and Collect Binge/Purge Log

The session starts with the therapist walking the patient to her office where she is weighed and asked how many times she has binged and purged in the past 7 days. Although these numbers are carefully noted on the therapist's binge/purge charts, these behaviors and these symptoms are largely under control at this point in treatment. Because treatment is at an advanced stage, more time is spent on general events of the past week or so. This brief period is still the only time the therapist meets with the adolescent without the rest of her family present, and it presents a crucial opportunity to continue to cultivate a relationship with her.

THERAPIST: How have things been the past few weeks?

LISA: I went to my cousin's gymnastics meet Saturday and that was so long—it was like, how long was it? It was almost 10 hours I was there.

THERAPIST: Wow. Did your whole family go?

LISA: No, it was just me, my aunt, and my cousins. Then Sunday it was my aunt's birthday, so we went out to dinner and that was nice. And I woke up almost everyday at 9.

THERAPIST: Wow! Keeping regular hours is good, and will help you eat regular meals at regular times.

LISA: Yeah, I did so well, it was only two times that I didn't wake up.

THERAPIST: Great, how were you able to do it?

LISA: Alarm.

THERAPIST: Did you get that new alarm clock?

LISA: No, no I used my old one.

THERAPIST: Uh-huh.

LISA: But, yeah, I wake up hungry. Most of the time I'd wake up at, like, 6:30, like I had this clock in me or something that wakes me up.

THERAPIST: So you're hungry when you wake up?

LISA: Yeah.

THERAPIST: Does that mean you're eating breakfast a little easier?

LISA: A little.

THERAPIST: Good. Did you eat breakfast each of the times you woke up?

LISA: Yes.

THERAPIST: Great! That's wonderful! So you're up to three meals?

LISA: Yeah.

THERAPIST: And any snack?

LISA: Yeah, I had graham crackers and something little in the evening.

THERAPIST: That sounds great.

LISA: Yeah.

THERAPIST: Congratulations!

LISA: Thanks.

THERAPIST: That's really a huge step. I know that it's been really hard to begin . . .

LISA: Yeah, well . . .

THERAPIST: Has your mom been helping you to wake up or have you been doing that on your own?

LISA: Sometimes. Not all the time, it's hard for me to sleep in, and if I'm waking up I don't want to stop.

THERAPIST: Uh-huh.

LISA: I go downstairs to eat breakfast. Well, I mean, I can't go to sleep again.

THERAPIST: Uh-huh. Great. Really wonderful. It seems like that was the last hurdle in regulating your eating and sleeping patterns.

LISA: Uh-huh.

THERAPIST: You've really been able to work hard on regulating your eating and sleeping patterns. Really wonderful, congratulations. What's happening in terms of bingeing and purging?

LISA: Uh, none.

THERAPIST: Congratulations! It's been 4 weeks now, and there hasn't been a binge or a purge.

LISA: Yeah.

THERAPIST: Wow. You're eating three meals, you got the snacks, it sounds like you're really doing a lot with that. Good. Do you want to take a look at weight?

LISA: Sure.

THERAPIST: What are you expecting?

LISA: Probably more, higher. Something more.

THERAPIST: Is that what you were expecting?

LISA: I don't know what it was before, so . . . I forgot.

THERAPIST: It was actually 121. We can fluctuate within a normal range, but recently there's been a little drop, to a lower rate. You started out at about 138 and now you're down to 126, about 12 pounds.

LISA: Okay.

THERAPIST: Why do you think there's been a shift in weight? I know you've gone up and down since then. Part of it is fluctuation, maybe part of it is due to something else?

LISA: About maybe digesting my food, and maybe my metabolism is working? I don't know.

THERAPIST: I think that's a reasonable explanation.

LISA: Uh-huh.

THERAPIST: Do you feel that your meals have been big and healthy?

LISA: Yeah, I feel full after I eat.

THERAPIST: Do you ever ignore intense hunger, or do you feel you're kind of snacking at mealtime instead of being a proper meal?

LISA: No, but twice I've had a meal at night because I didn't during the day.

THERAPIST: So you compensated for not eating earlier in the day?

LISA: Yeah, I compensated.

THERAPIST: Well, good, that's great. All right, I'm going to go get your parents. Is there anything that you want to talk about before we bring them in?

LISA: No.

THERAPIST: Anything around any meals that you want to bring up?

LISA: No.

THERAPIST: Okay.

After about 5 or 10 minutes of conversation, the therapist asks the rest of the family to join them in the office. The therapist would typically start this part of the meeting by sharing her binge/purge charts with the parents to reconcile the patient's report with the parents' impressions of how the week has gone. As noted, less time is usually spent lingering over this report at this stage of treatment, because the patient is progressing well and eating is mostly under her control.

Continue to Support and Assist Parents in Management of Eating Disorder Symptoms until the Adolescent Is Able to Eat Well on Her Own without Binge Eating and Purging

THERAPIST: So your impression is that things have been going quite well?

MOTHER: Very good. We're at the top of the mountain now, having fun.

THERAPIST: What did you specifically notice at home since our last meeting?

MOTHER: She seems to be eating later into the night, and more or less back to cereal or granola, and once in a while meat loaf or a hamburger, which she would normally barely eat.

LISA: No, I didn't eat hamburger, I had meat loaf.

THERAPIST: Okay.

MOTHER: I think she's feeling better in general.

THERAPIST: Well you've noticed her eating a larger variety of food.

MOTHER: Yes.

THERAPIST: She's waking up earlier, and that means that she's eating breakfast.

MOTHER: Right.

THERAPIST: And she's been hungry at breakfast too?

MOTHER: Yeah, she's been hungry a lot. I mean, she's not going for the apple, she's going for a bowl of oatmeal or something, without me even suggesting it, so you know she's really getting better.

THERAPIST: So some of the things that you planned, in terms of getting Lisa up in the morning, like setting the alarm, worked?

MOTHER: Yes. I think it was just her setting her mind to it, that she had to do it. That really worked. You're feeling better, aren't you?

LISA: Yeah.

MOTHER: Because you have set your alarm, you have done it. It took some time for us to figure it out, but now we know better how to balance the sleeping and eating times.

THERAPIST: I think you guys did it. I think a lot of that session was focused on, "What really do I do," in terms of planning and how do you go about telling her.

MOTHER: Yeah. She's sleeping better, I think, at night.

LISA: I'm definitely sleeping.

THERAPIST: Uh-huh.

FATHER: Yeah she goes right to sleep.

MOTHER: Uh-huh.

In the exchange above the therapist was inquiring about the level of difficulty Lisa was having with eating under parental control without resorting
to binge eating and purging. The tone of the session is positive and optimistic because Lisa's progress has been excellent.

Assist Parents and Adolescent in Negotiating the Return of Control of Eating-Related Behaviors to the Adolescent

THERAPIST: I really think that getting your sleeping and eating worked out
was the biggest and last hurdle to get over, because for some time now
the bingeing and purging has been under control. Right from the start
you, the family, have really been able to work at incorporating new
foods into Lisa's diet, and she's been able to keep doing that well on
her own, if I'm not mistaken.

MOTHER: Uh-huh.

THERAPIST: So it sounds like the things you've been doing in the past, like
monitoring meals and monitoring Lisa after meals, has really helped
with the bingeing and purging. There has been no bingeing and purging or any symptoms for about a month now. That's wonderful. And
you're making sure you're getting your meals?

MOTHER: Yes. She seems to be exercising more too.

FATHER: Yeah.

MOTHER: Which I think has helped probably with the sleep.

THERAPIST: Well, we talked a little last time about how to get some exercise
going. (to Lisa) Did your [parents] help you with the exercise? What
did your mom do?

LISA: Well, the first day we went walking, but that's about it.

MOTHER: Lisa's been working out down in the basement pretty much.

FATHER: That's been helpful, I think.

THERAPIST: Do you think Lisa's been doing a lot of these things on her
own? Or is it because you've been helping her?

MOTHER: Definitely on her own.

FATHER: Yeah.

MOTHER: I think she feels a little bit more independent again, like she used
to. I really do. She includes me in on a lot of things, but it seems like
she's getting a little more independent, I suppose, which is a great feeling for all of us.

THERAPIST: In what ways have you seen Lisa become more independent?

FATHER: Well, she's more willing to go out, like with this trip. And she's taking the initiative.

THERAPIST: So there's less of the two of you helping her through activities and more of her taking the initiative?

MOTHER: Definitely.

FATHER: Oh, yeah.

THERAPIST: (to Lisa) Would you agree? What about some of the things your parents have said?

LISA: Yeah. My dad helps with planning my exercise routine, so I don't overdo it.

THERAPIST: And that helps?

LISA: I don't really need help any more, I don't think.

THERAPIST: So that's just sort of a normal thing your dad does to help you out, but not specifically around eating?

LISA: Yeah.

THERAPIST: Okay.

THERAPIST: So it seems things are going much better. It's been kind of a natural progression, you've backed off, and you did so even before we started talking about it. I think that's worked out quite well. (to Lisa) And you've responded quite well.

MOTHER: (to Lisa) I think you're ready to feel better, aren't you?

LISA: Yeah.

MOTHER: We'll see how this next week goes, when she's away from us and having fun with her cousins.

THERAPIST: It sounds like that will be a great opportunity to really test her independence.

MOTHER: It really will. She won't be staying with my mother-in-law. She'll be staying in a condo right there in the complex, so they're going to take care of themselves food-wise pretty much. She'll have a lot of independent time where she's going have to take care of herself and make sure she takes her Lexapro and makes sure she eats.

THERAPIST: How have things with the Lexapro been going?

MOTHER: Good. You know, she's just taking 5 mg, which seems to be enough for her. She just doesn't feel like she needs more, and why give it to her if she doesn't?

In this exchange the therapist is exploring the parents' sense of Lisa's readiness for managing her eating behavior with less of their consistent monitoring. In this instance the parents have already been testing the waters a bit on Lisa's ability to be more independent and have a plan to test her ability with a trip to relatives. The therapist is comfortable with this decision because all indications are that the parents' plan is reasonable. Should the therapist be concerned, closer questioning of the decision would have been likely, though without undermining the parents' decision making.

Encourage Family Members to Examine Relationships between Adolescent Issues and the Development of BN in Their Adolescent

THERAPIST: I think right now, we're at the end of Stage 2. Stage 1 was focused on having you guys involved in curtailing the bingeing and purging, specifically the purging, and also trying to increase the variety of foods, making sure that Lisa is getting in proper meals and snacks. I think that all of you did a wonderful job with that. Stage 2 is focused on handing control of these issues back to Lisa. And it sounds like that is happening. Even in this process things have continued to go even better, in terms of food, because you've been able to add in breakfast. And it sounds like we're at this end of Stage 2 where things are back in Lisa's control. (*to Lisa*) You're going off next week, you're on your own, and it sounds like it's going quite well. Do you agree with that?

LISA: Yeah.

MOTHER: I think it was good that we realized that she needed to sit and eat dinner with us. I think, as a bulimic, it is not an easy thing to do. She would pull away or just prefer to be by herself. When she sat at the dinner table, she interacted with us, ate with us. I think it was a big step in helping her because she hadn't eaten with us in a while.

FATHER: You know she wants to, though.

THERAPIST: And what are the family meals like now?

FATHER: Family meals? It's the same empty talk, I'm afraid. (*laughing*)

MOTHER: Yeah, she's been eating with us more.

THERAPIST: That's a start.

MOTHER: Then she'll still make sure she saves enough—she'll take a little bit "for the road." And she'll sit at the table and do that, I'll be in the kitchen, and if any of us get up early from the table . . .

FATHER: Oh, she starts . . . we have to stay till she finishes.

MOTHER: She says, "I am not finished yet."

THERAPIST: Your husband and son just get up and leave?

MOTHER: Well, when they're done—they don't like to sit.

THERAPIST: So how do you decide on your meal choices? How about that?

MOTHER: I think that's mostly up to me. You know, I pretty much know what everyone likes and how they like to have it. It's pretty much up to me.

THERAPIST: So is everyone eating the same thing?

MOTHER: Yes, pretty much.

THERAPIST: So you're eating most meals together?

LISA: Uh-huh.

THERAPIST: And you're eating the same things?

MOTHER: Yeah, salad . . . vegetables.

THERAPIST: And you've been preparing all the meals?

MOTHER: Pretty much. Lisa likes to cook a little bit, you know, she'll prepare some things.

THERAPIST: Is that true?

LISA: Yeah.

MOTHER: Yeah she'll do a vegetable or the main course or something.

THERAPIST: (to Lisa) Do you have any input on what goes into the meals?

LISA: Well, yeah, she'll ask me what we should have for dinner.

MOTHER: Sometimes we go online. We made chicken scallopini one night and stew another night.

THERAPIST: And do you go grocery shopping?

MOTHER: Most of the time I go by myself. But I usually ask her if there's anything she wants.

THERAPIST: And are you all right with this . . . arrangement?

LISA: I'm comfortable.

THERAPIST: And you play some role in choosing some of the food and some of the preparation too?

LISA: Yeah.

THERAPIST: Okay.

MOTHER: Even if I wasn't around, she'd do it. You know, if I was gone for the day or something, she would cook something so she'd have something for the day. She does for the first two meals anyway.

THERAPIST: Right. So the first two meals, what happens?

LISA: One I eat salad, and one I eat vegetables.

MOTHER: But before 9 P.M..

THERAPIST: And you're not eating breakfast with her?

MOTHER: No. . .

THERAPIST: And lunch, where are you eating specifically?

MOTHER: At home most of the time.

THERAPIST: And portions, how do you end up deciding the portions? Do you do this on your own?

LISA: Well, it depends if I'm full.

THERAPIST: Is this for dinner? Is this dishing out food yourself or does one person dish the food?

MOTHER: Is this good or bad? We just take what we think we can eat.

THERAPIST: Every family is very different.

MOTHER: Yeah.

THERAPIST: It's appropriate at this stage for Lisa to dish up her own food.

MOTHER: She knows what she can eat and what she can't.

THERAPIST: I get the perspective that things are going well. You're starting again to socialize, which I think is very big step, and it's a wonderful indicator of your great progress. Any other plans, what are you doing? I know you're going away next week. What are some of your plans after that?

LISA: I don't have any plans at all. I mean, I can't stay at home next fall.

FATHER: Good . . . I mean really. We would like her to be in a safe school for 1 year and then if she wants to go to a college within a couple of hours, she can do that . . .

MOTHER: . . . as long as we can get to her if she has any problem related to the BN.

FATHER: The challenge is to make good choices along the way.

THERAPIST: And how does Lisa feel about this?

FATHER: Well, she wants to go further. She's not happy with her school choices. But we would like to see her stay nearby . . .

MOTHER: . . . even if it was for 6 months, till January or February, just so we feel comfortable and she feels comfortable. But she puts an awful lot of pressure on herself when it comes to academics, and we've got to be close to support her a little bit.

FATHER: If that works, then she'll be pushing along to go to another school of her choice.

MOTHER: Or she could even transfer spring semester—that would be great.

THERAPIST: It sounds like the two of you are on the same page.

FATHER: We are.

MOTHER: We just don't know what she wants yet. We'll see how she does this next week when she's gone.

FATHER: Well, you don't necessarily have to go to college.

LISA: Yes, Dad, I do.

MOTHER: Well, I don't know. We could look into something else if you were interested—for example, fashion, or something that interests you but doesn't require college. Some people don't want to go to college. You are so interested in history that I think it's a good thing, which is a nice fall back.

FATHER: You can do anything you want.

THERAPIST: Lisa, what's your response after hearing that?

LISA: I don't care, but I want to learn more.

THERAPIST: You see now what you don't want to do (stay at home).

LISA: Yeah.

THERAPIST: You've been clear on what you don't want to do?

LISA: It's all the same, I mean . . . (laughter)

FATHER: 'Cause if you want to go away to college, you'd better tell us where you want to go, because you have to let us know. You can't just tell us at the last minute.

THERAPIST: Have you thought about that?

FATHER: This isn't high school, so . . .

LISA: Well, I just don't know what I want to do.

In these exchanges the therapist is beginning to encourage the family to help Lisa resume her usual social life, which has been disrupted by the need to deal with her eating disorder. The therapist aims to put the issue of Lisa's social life on the agenda during the early sessions in Phase II, but not to examine it closely necessarily. The therapist will explore it more as Phase II progresses.

Assist Parents and Adolescent in Negotiating the Return of Control over Eating to the Adolescent

THERAPIST: Lisa's increasing independence is a difficult thing to try and negotiate at this early stage. Each family finds a different way to collaborate and figure out what stage is next because eating disorders really disrupt a lot of normal activities. It's therefore important at this stage for Lisa to get involved in a variety of age-appropriate activities. Lisa, you're starting to really get involved by going away, spending time with friends, and socializing much more. I know we've talked about it in several sessions, in terms of planning ahead and what you take from here. I think each family finds a different way of coming to that agreement of what comes next and I think it's the place of the family to be able to figure that out, but sometimes it's quite hard. You've negotiated on a lot of different fronts: First on the eating front, around bingeing and purging, finding ways to monitor the eating without making it too intrusive. You've negotiated on how to give the control back to Lisa, and this issue of college is the next hurdle right now.

MOTHER: We need to make her feel comfortable somewhere, and if she feels comfortable and we're comfortable with her, then she'll do okay.

FATHER: I think we should make a list of the places you want to go.

THERAPIST: What I see you guys doing so well is working through making difficult decisions. You as parents provided a whole slew of different options for Lisa in helping her make new choices about food and eating. Remember back then, in the very beginning, when we were talking about eating disorders and trying to find ways to increase Lisa's meal consumption and make sure they were healthy, nutritious meals? A lot of the options presented at first were not perfect, but you guys found a really wonderful way of moving things forward. A couple of suggestions I hear you talking about sound like really great ways of making the right choices.

FATHER: Well, we're here to help her with anything she wants to do.

THERAPIST: How do you feel about that?

LISA: Okay.

MOTHER: We have to know what you're thinking and then we'll try to help you get there.

FATHER: And stay away from Tucson [referring to traveling or college options]. Okay, you can put it on the list, somewhere way down the list (*jokingly*).

MOTHER: We're going to make that list. You could even go to Orland Park. There's a lot of options out there, you just have to realize they're there. I think we're good at recognizing options.

THERAPIST: I think you're excellent at that. I think you've all played a really significant role in being able to negotiate. I think it's your sensitivity toward each other that is so meaningful. It was very clear, even from the beginning, that you're very good at getting along with each other. Particularly as parents, you have a very good understanding of your daughter and what she needs in order to move forward and how you can support her to do that.

MOTHER: Well, we were awfully confused for a while. John and I were at our wit's end.

FATHER: One year ago we were in terrible shape.

MOTHER: We really were.

THERAPIST: And that's what happens. The eating disorder will come in and make you feel as if you don't know what you're doing.

MOTHER: It's horrible.

THERAPIST: Uh-huh. It's important to move on, to continue giving control back to Lisa and figuring out what the next step is. The final stage of therapy focuses on adolescent issues and different things that have gone on that you feel the eating disorder has interfered with. I'm going to start off by reviewing a little bit of what adolescent development is, and we'll talk a little bit more next session about that. Then we'll focus the last four sessions on whatever issues you feel are important. Right now we're at Session 15, but I think things have been progressing so well that we may not have to do the full 20?

FATHER: Please, we'd prefer to do the full 20.

MOTHER: No one's in a hurry.

FATHER: The thought occurred to me, what if things go bad or something happens? Then what do we do about it?

THERAPIST: Well, what's the answer to that?

FATHER: I don't know.

MOTHER: Did you keep up with eating well?

THERAPIST: I think it's very common for parents to feel that way, and it's a problem for many people toward the end of treatment.

MOTHER: I think she's realizing, though, that she's not going to gain weight by eating regular meals. Correct me if I'm wrong, Lisa. She's eating a lot of things, even a little ice cream or some other dessert. Some weeks she'll lose a pound or 2 and then stay level. You know, she's staying right at a certain limit.

THERAPIST: Yes, she's eating regular meals and maintaining a healthy weight.

MOTHER: Like a normal person. I hope she knows she can beat this eating disorder. I don't know, I don't know if when she gets away and around people who . . . I don't know . . . I think, when I'm not there, it's going to be different.

LISA: People who are thinner? Is that what you mean?

MOTHER: No, I mean people who don't eat or eat fast food types of things.

In this exchange the therapist uses externalization to help the family see how much BN had disrupted their lives as well as Lisa's. The therapist also discusses the usefulness of negotiating the changes with Lisa while still ensuring that the parents understood their responsibility. Negotiation with the adolescent with BN occurs much more often than with the adolescent with anorexia in both Phase I and II. Negotiation is one of the ways to broach differences between the adolescent and parents that minimizes tension and criticism.

Close Sessions with Positive Support

THERAPIST: I think we'll focus more and more on that issue in the later stages. I think one really important point to keep in mind is to realize the extent of what you've done in terms of this treatment. I've merely been a facilitator as this process has been going on in your family. From the beginning you're the ones who've done everything. When you came in, you realized there was a problem. You took Lisa out of school and ended up getting her into treatment right away. Throughout this treatment you've played the active role, as a team. I think that that's really the key to what makes this treatment successful at overcoming an eating disorder.

MOTHER: But the question is, when she moves out . . . then what?

THERAPIST: Right.

MOTHER: Can she manage to eat right out there, with no nearby support from us?

THERAPIST: (to Lisa) What's your response?

LISA: Totally.

FATHER: Well, *totally* for right now, but she has 5 more months to solidify her progress before she moves out.

MOTHER: Right and she's got to realize we're still there for the support.

FATHER: And we just want to make sure we're close to her.

THERAPIST: You've noticed some major changes in terms of the way that Lisa's been thinking. You're talking about clarifying her thinking more. Yes, you do still have time to solidify a lot of those gains. But to a certain degree, you've seen that happen already. From the start Lisa has shown a shift in attitude that's only increased since then, and I think that progress is important to keep in mind. Here you're also talking about not being that far away from her so that you can provide support physically, but also you're plugged into what's going on in Lisa's life. So you want to move from that perspective.

FATHER: That's right.

MOTHER: I think she's ready to move on and not have us so close. You know to be . . . it's difficult when she has people wondering, we're there, you know where she can have someone come into a dorm room or something and clean up the house with guys, having to take a shower without much privacy, roommates going back and forth. They're 19, 20 years old, you know, you could tell it's extremely awkward for her.

THERAPIST: And this living arrangement is not going to work?

MOTHER: It's time to, yeah, and I think she really misses school.

THERAPIST: And you want to assist her to get back into that world?

MOTHER: Right, you have to take a chance, you know, and she's just gotta know we're there.

THERAPIST: You're doing a great, great job, all of you. I know I've said this quite few times, but I am thoroughly impressed with you, as a family, to be able to do this so quickly, so efficiently. You have a very good understanding of what we're dealing with here. And you've done, really, such a great job on your own in terms of giving 100% of yourselves.

MOTHER: Thanks.

FATHER: Thanks.

MOTHER: Someone told me about a mother whose daughter had BN. The mom talked about how you think about it all the time, you think about if she's getting better, until all of a sudden you just completely forget that she ever had BN. I can't wait till then. (*laughing*)

THERAPIST: What stage are you in?

MOTHER: We think about it a lot less, I kind of forget about it.

The therapist closes the session with enthusiasm and optimism. The brief review serves as a kind of coda for this first session of Phase II: It demarcates the work that has preceded and anticipates the work ahead. The following chapter outlines the goals and interventions for Phase III and concludes with a final example of a session in action.

CHAPTER 12

Phase III

*Adolescent Developmental Concerns
(Sessions 17–20)*

In this chapter we discuss the goals, interventions, and timing of Phase III. The therapist can anticipate possibly spending more time in this phase than the allotted four sessions, especially in those cases where progression from Phase I to II was relatively smooth and brief. However, we usually assume that Phase III does not constitute a resolution of adolescent issues, per se, but rather a discussion of these family-specific issues in three to five sessions. The goal is to set family members on a course that would enable them to resolve these issues as they arise. In this chapter we also present a general discussion of adolescent development in relation to the eating disorder to serve as an introduction to the overall types of issues that are addressed in this phase. Finally, we focus on how termination is managed in this type of therapy.

The third phase is initiated when the patient's bulimic symptoms are absent, caloric restriction has abated and weight is stable, and decision making around eating is firmly within the adolescent's domain. In other words, the parents as well as the adolescent feel comfortable about the teen's control over what, when, or whether she eats. This evaluation is dependent on the age of the adolescent as well as the specific rules and habits around eating of each particular family. The central goal in this phase is to foster a healthy adolescent–parent relationship in which the illness does not constitute the basis of interaction. This goal entails, among other things, working toward appropriate intergenerational boundaries and the need for the parents to reorganize their life as a couple in light of their children's prospective departure. Attention to parental professional and leisure interests are a legitimate focus of this phase. Unlike the case of AN, most adolescents with BN are age appropriately independent, so relatively less focus is placed on the issue of personal autonomy.

At this point in treatment a discussion of adolescent issues such as leaving home, independence, and sexuality may be conducted because the adolescent–parent relationship is no longer entangled in the eating disorder. Each family will present with its unique issues, and the therapist should let the family take the lead in determining which issues are discussed in sessions. The therapist commonly helps parents recognize that they can have personal priorities—that they can seek their own paths as a couple and as individuals—and that their children will increasingly play a different role in their lives. These final sessions are not supposed to resolve these matters; instead, they are designed to help the parents communicate to their children that these matters are the parents' concern and they, as a couple, will attend to them.

Readiness for Phase III

Phase III is a brief phase characterized by the conviction that the bulimic symptoms are largely absent and that there is a strong likelihood that they will not recur; therefore, the symptoms cease to be the focus of discussion. However, the concern that the eating disorder may resurface is addressed. In addition, although the patient may still be somewhat preoccupied with worries about weight and shape, a discussion of these concerns is less fraught with anxiety. As noted above, an adolescent is ready for Phase III when bulimic symptoms are absent, weight is within a normal range (if this was a concern), and responsibility for healthy eating has been handed back to the patient, as is appropriate given her age. The adolescent–parent relationship is no longer focused on the symptomatic behaviors, and a discussion of general adolescent developmental issues (e.g., leaving home, independence, sexuality) may now be conducted.

The technique employed in these sessions builds on the increasing autonomy of the patient and her parents from the therapist, which has evolved during the previous two phases of treatment. That is, meetings with the therapist are spaced at greater intervals (3–4 weeks apart) and the family is expected to be better able to take on general challenges of adolescence than when the symptomatic expressions of BN dominated the daily life. In this sense, the family and the patient are ready to take on the issues of adolescence as a developmental process, supporting the ultimate autonomy and emancipation of the adolescent from the control of the parents.

Building on the more optimistic mood in Phase II, the family often feels increased energy and interest in taking on the more general issues of adolescence that often feel easier to manage compared to BN. Because of their successful efforts at helping their daughter reestablish healthy eating, the family can now be hopeful about her success in adolescence. This is not to say that there will not be a sense of loss about the change of status of their daughter from child to young adult; in fact, this loss may indeed be one of the themes that will need to be explored. The brighter mood of these sessions, however, supports the family's competence to take on the continuing challenges of adolescence.

Throughout this treatment the therapist has maintained a supportive stance toward the adolescent while carefully separating her from the symptomatic expression of BN. Particularly in this phase, the therapist provides ample support for her growing need for deserved autonomy. The therapist's task is made a little easier if he/she has succeeded in *not* alienating the patient in the earlier phases. This point underscores the need to avoid focusing solely on the parents alone during those early sessions, but to consider the adolescent as an active participant in her own recovery. For this last phase to work, it is important for the therapist to continue to enhance the earlier alliance.

Finally, this brief phase can accommodate a direct discussion of only a few major issues or challenges, such as dating, leaving home, or choosing a college. This time limitation encourages the family and therapist to prioritize the most important issues to work on during sessions, while acknowledging other issues that may be considered by the family outside of the sessions. In this sense, this phase constitutes targeted family therapy for adolescents who have recovered from an eating disorder.

As is the case in moving from Phase I to II and again from Phase II to III, the therapist announces the transition to the family; in other words, she/he lets the family know when sufficient progress has been made to "graduate" to the next phase of treatment. When the adolescent and her parents move from Phase II to III, the therapist will briefly summarize the main points of this last phase. In particular, the therapist will make it clear, especially to the adolescent, that reviewing bulimic symptoms and weighing the patient are not considered core features of this phase because it is assumed that these concerns are no longer central to the therapy.

The major goals for this phase of treatment are:

- To establish that the adolescent–parent relationship is no longer defined by BN symptoms.
- To review adolescent developmental tasks with the family.
- To terminate treatment.

In order to accomplish these goals, the therapist should undertake the following interventions:

1. Review adolescent issues with family and model problem solving of these issues.
2. Involve family in review of adolescent issues.
3. Delineate and explore adolescent themes.
4. Ask parents about how much they are doing as a couple, separate from their children.
5. Prepare for challenges and issues that may arise in the future.
6. Terminate treatment.

Adolescent Development and BN

Phase III of FBT for BN is structurally very similar to that used in AN, except that the therapist usually works on earlier adolescent issues with patients with AN than is the case in adolescent BN. Many adolescents with BN enter the latter stages of adolescence as they approach the completion of treatment (see below for a review of stages of adolescence). For example, planning for college and careers and gaining skills for more meaningful interpersonal relationships outside the family may be topics ripe for discussion during these final sessions. In general, this stage is characterized by increased wishes for emotional and sexual intimacy with peers, and less need for a familial base of support. Challenges that might arise in this phase of treatment are derived from residual problems in areas such as continued excessive emotional or physical dependency on parents or family, continued anxiety about body image, sex, and intimacy. All of these issues can be adversely affected by BN. For instance, an adolescent with BN may be especially reluctant to share her body with a romantic partner because of fears surrounding the acceptability of her body shape. FBT is especially important in helping parents who may be anxious about supporting their daughter's development of romantic relationships or who may prevent the exploration of career or educational opportunities that take the adolescent away from home. Parents, too, must accomplish developmental tasks associated with the adolescent process in their children. Following are some suggestions that may help parents during this transitional phase of treatment:

- Develop activities, interests, and skills that constitute a postparenting life (i.e., involve only the couple).
- Develop an identity as a couple (i.e., one that is not defined solely by being parents).
- Discover ways in which parental roles, work, leisure interests, and studies can be integrated with the interests and needs of the developing adults in the household.
- Accept the distinctive physical and emotional aspects of sexual development, orientation, and interests of growing adolescents.
- Give up the skills, attitudes, and activities that were appropriate to earlier developmental stages of children.
- Evolve personal capacities that increase the adolescents' ability to see and accept parents as developing individuals.

Each of these topics may be a theme in the third phase of treatment. The failure of parents to accomplish these tasks may make it more difficult for the adolescent to complete her own transition to adulthood. Therapists may use this list as a way to identify a specific focus for the interventions with the couple that are used during this treatment phase.

Teamwork in Phase III

Teamwork will likely have evolved from Phase I to Phase III in that there will be a decrease in involvement with team members who are outside the primary therapeutic intervention. Usually, by the time a patient reaches Phase III with success, the pediatrician has long since decreased monitoring the patient because the documented progress is such that the adolescent is medically safe. However, it is likely (and should be encouraged) that the patient continues to maintain these relationships at least until the conclusion of therapy. The relationship among the therapeutic team members (e.g., cotherapist who treats a comorbid condition) remains as active and important as before. As family members move toward termination, they may attempt to involve one or both of the therapists in family dynamics to undermine this process. Likewise, termination may also be difficult for therapists who have invested in the recovery of this patient and family. The therapeutic team can help identify these issues more clearly, so that they can be approached systematically.

Review Adolescent Issues with the Family and Model Problem Solving of These Types of Issues

Why

Because many young patients with BN develop difficulties in negotiating general adolescent developmental issues, it is important to assist them and their parents in reintegrating the patients *into adolescence* after bulimic symptoms have abated. In rare instances (in contrast to AN patients) of debilitating bulimic symptoms, the adolescent with BN might be required to be absent from school for periods of time. In such instances she might remain dependent on her parents because of the behavioral, psychological, and medical needs that are associated with overcoming BN. Because of her battle with BN over a period of months or even years, the adolescent may not be entirely in sync with her peers. Upon cessation of bulimic symptoms, these other issues may need to be addressed. A large range of needs in this area should be expected, and successful resolution will depend on the resources of the individual patient and those that her family brings to bear on the problems. For example, in a relatively uncomplicated case where the establishment of healthy eating was achieved with little difficulty and there are generally few problematic issues in the family, getting the adolescent back on track may be fairly straightforward. On the other hand, when the reestablishment of healthy eating in Phases I and II did not proceed smoothly or has been complicated by a comorbid psychiatric illness, and/or other family or individual problems, more work on problem solving around these specific comorbid issues and how these may impact ongoing adolescent development may be required in Phase III. During this final phase, the patient's anger about how she has been treated during the process to reestablish healthy eating also may become a focus. It is helpful for parents to acknowledge what they can do about the daughter's complaints regarding what she may feel was taken from her. It must be emphasized that the approach described here is more applicable to patients who have less complicated cases and their healthy eating has been firmly reestablished by Phase III. An additional course of adolescent family psychotherapy may well be required in very complex cases, and the issues that need to be addressed in such instances may go well beyond the outlines provided in this manual.

How

The therapist should begin this phase by reviewing the progress the patient and her parents have made together thus far. In this way the therapist should bring to light the pertinent challenges that were identified by the therapist, the adolescent, or her parents earlier in treatment. These are the issues that were deferred in order to focus on getting the unhealthy eating behavior out of the way. By orienting the parents to the topic of adolescent development, the therapist can identify a range of themes to consider and help ensure that most relevant challenges are included for this discussion. More emotionally charged issues, such as sexual development and behavior, might need special emphasis if the family attempts to avoid these. In this part of treatment, it is not uncommon for the therapist to deliver this message in what appears to be somewhat of a monologue.

Involve Parents in Review of Adolescent Issues

Why

Involving the parents in the review of adolescent issues, as these relate to their child's development, helps the parents and the adolescent identify and specify areas of concern. It allows the parents to demonstrate that their skill-set in helping the adolescent through her bulimia will be helpful in other non-eating disorder issues. Involving the parents in this way also helps the adolescent, with the support of the therapist, to guide the parents in just how much they ought to be involved given adolescent's age and this late stage of treatment. It also helps to reinforce, by repetition and making the information more personally relevant, the content of the mini-lecture on adolescent development that the therapist just delivered.

How

As discussed at the end of Phase II, the therapist and family can now address some of the identified issues of adolescence. For example, the therapist might mention that early on in treatment, the patient complained about how her parents seldom allowed her to make her own decisions "about just everything." At that point in the treatment, the therapist did not ask the adolescent to elaborate in too much detail. However, Phase III is the appropriate time to examine these issues more thoroughly. For instance, the therapist might ask the adolescent:

> "Let's talk a little bit more about your feeling that your parents do not allow you to make many, or any, of your own decisions. Can you tell me a little more about that?"

Likewise, the parents may be asked to give their thoughts on what their daughter has said and also state their views regarding decision making in their family. Such a discussion gives the therapist an opportunity to help the family explore the issue of decision making and age-appropriate autonomy and how to arrive at a resolution of such dilemmas. It is helpful if the therapist is able to identify issues raised by all family members. To do this requires that the therapist be alert to potential Phase III issues from the start of the treatment process, and to keep a record of these so that they can be used as concrete examples in Phase III. It is important that the therapist enable the parents and the adolescent to come to agreement on the particular issues of adolescent development (e.g., dating, time away from the family, leaving home). This discussion is akin to the strategy employed in Phase I of empowering the parents, in collaboration with the adolescent, to deal with BN. The aim here is to engage the parents and the patient in a discussion of the process of adolescence, and to encourage them to approach and deal with these problems as they see fit and as applicable to their own family.

After a number of these key issues have been identified, it is sometimes helpful for the therapist to spend a few minutes providing an overview of the types of issues that all families with teenagers are likely to encounter, such as staying out past a curfew, being caught drinking alcohol, experimenting with recreational drugs, or telling their parents that they have sex with their partner. This overview helps to normalize the process of adolescence for the patient and the family as well as provide an opportunity to educate the family about this general process. Next, the therapist should attempt to integrate the issues identified by the patient and her parents into the overall scheme of adolescent development that was presented. This should be an interactive process that involves the parents in incorporating their own past issues into the overall adolescent developmental scheme. For instance, the therapist should ask the parents to talk about their own experiences during adolescence. Recognition of the challenges they themselves faced during their adolescence might help them better understand their daughter's struggles. The therapist should provide guidance in this process but should allow most of the discussion to come from the adolescent and her parents.

Delineate and Explore Adolescent Themes

Why

In order to help the parents find ways to manage the adolescent process now that the BN behavior is behind them, the therapist should provide targeted assistance in problem solving that may serve as a template for their efforts at home after completion of therapy. It is important for the parents and the adolescent to explore some of the issues of adolescence without the eating problems interfering or becoming the focus of their communication. Family members need to appreciate that they do have the skills to manage more general issues now that the eating disorder is no longer present.

How

This task of delineating and exploring adolescent themes can be achieved using the circular questioning strategy employed in earlier sessions. This technique involves the whole family and helps to "flesh out" the issues. Sufficient detail about the problem must be evident to provide the therapist with material for interpretation. By this point, of course, the therapist will have a sophisticated understanding of how this family is likely to approach (or not approach) certain problematic issues. This knowledge provides a considerable advantage because the way the family managed the problem with eating and weight is likely to be similar to how it may manage other problems of adolescence. For example, if a theme identified for the patient is her need for support in the development of friendships, the therapist might begin by asking each parent for his/her view on the importance of friends outside the family. Next the therapist might ask the adolescent whether she agrees with her parents' view and if she feels supported by her parents in developing friendships. If there are other adolescent family members, their views should also be solicited. As family members describe their thoughts and experiences, the therapist should be prepared to provide assistance when there are problems. If, for example, it is clear that the parents are overly restrictive, the therapist should ask the parents why they feel this need to restrict their daughter and what would make them more open to her developing friendships outside the family. A dialogue should ensue that allows the therapist, patient, and parents to come to an agreement about how best to make friendships more available within the context of the parental concerns.

Ask Parents How Much They Are Doing as a Couple, Separate from Their Children

Why

It is important that parents also successfully nurture their own relationship now that the immediate crisis of the eating disorder has passed. Much of the therapy has encouraged joint parental action in the face of the difficulties of their daughter's BN, which might have become the main way the couple has related to one another for some time. However, in order to support both the increased appropriate autonomy of their daughter and their own relationship, the therapist's focus on the parents' needs and their relationship is warranted.

This therapy and this phase of treatment, in particular, is not an attempt at an abbreviated treatment for the couple any more than it is an attempt to complete a full-fledged family therapy for emerging adolescents. Instead, the idea is to identify the need for the couple to consider their own relationship and its needs in the changed context of their daughter's renewed health and ongoing successful adolescent development. Modest expectations should be set if the therapist considers it appropriate and necessary to address the parents' relationship, especially if there are major relationship problems between the spouses. This intervention should not constitute couple therapy if such therapy is needed to address the major problems in the relationship. However, in many cases, the eating disorder and its treatment are the source of any derailment in the parental dyad. In these cases, simply indicating that there is a potential problem that may need to be addressed is sufficient to set things on the right course. On the other hand, parental difficulties that predate the eating disorder may have been put aside in the interest of their daughter's health. These problems may reemerge at this juncture, but the treatment in this manual will likely not address these types of problems. Instead, the couple may seek additional treatment elsewhere, and the therapist should help facilitate this referral.

How

In order to accomplish this treatment goal, the therapist should ask the parents how much time they spend together, what they do, and how this pattern compares to their experiences of one another prior to the onset of the BN. The therapist does not need to intervene with specific ideas about how to improve this relationship structure; instead she/he should encourage the exploration of these issues between the partners themselves. The therapist should make it clear that this is not a shift to couple therapy, only an attempt to encourage the partners to think more about their own relationship and how they, as a couple, spend time together. If this discussion devolves into major discord between the parents, the therapist will, of course, intervene and provide them with an appropriate referral for couple counseling.

Preparing for Future Issues

Why

In order to support the family, it is important for the therapist to help members find ways to cope with future dilemmas or challenges. This effort by the therapist helps to communicate continuing investment in the family and also specific ways to proceed if problems occur.

How

The therapist can provide some guidance about what kinds of issues the future might hold; for example, the patient leaving for college or work, different ways in which the parents might help facilitate this step for the adolescent, targeted issues (e.g., overly close attachment to a parent, or parents' concern about friends patient is associating with) for which there was no time to explore in this treatment setting, and so forth. Again, the therapist should be alert to the time and emphasis placed on this therapeutic maneuver—this is a brief phase of treatment and a review of adolescent developmental issues should take precedence over other issues. Consequently, no more than a session ought to be spent on this particular therapeutic intervention. It is important that all family members have an opportunity to participate and be involved in this discussion, so the therapist should direct the conversation in such a way that every family member present has an opportunity to voice an opinion about how to cope with future dilemmas when they arise. It is also likely that the patient and parental issues may dominate the discussion, as was the case during the earlier session in this phase, though perhaps less so.

Terminate Treatment

Why

As important as greeting the family at the outset of treatment was, so is the process of a respectful conclusion of the treatment. This process should clearly end the therapeutic relationship by conferring on the adolescent and her parents the sincere confidence that they can proceed with likely success if future problems arise. FBT for adolescents using the family model described in this manual lasts approximately 6 months. Although the early interventions of this treatment are the most intense and most closely spaced, the involvement with the family, albeit less frequent, is still significant and meaningful in this latter part of treatment. The early use of the authority of the therapist to engage the family in the seriousness of the illness makes the relationship with the therapist an intense one. During Phases II and III great effort is made to decrease the dependence on the therapist while also increasing both the patient's and the family's autonomous functioning in line with the ultimate goal of a successful termination. The method of termination employed here is not necessarily specific, but the key concern is that the family has an opportunity to review the therapy, discuss relapse prevention, and say goodbye to the therapist, and the therapist has an opportunity to convey optimism and support in the process of separation.

How

At the final treatment session, the therapist should reserve about half the time to conclude the therapy by saying goodbye to each family member. This termination ritual should mirror the first session's momentous and careful greeting of each family member. Attention should be paid to each family member's involvement, with ample praise for the work done on behalf of the family. A genuine warmth, a comforting quality, as well as a subdued optimism should characterize the therapist's demeanor. Family members should each be given an opportunity to bid the therapist farewell. The therapist's aim is to encourage the family's abilities to proceed smoothly and undertake successfully any problems that are ahead.

    The principal method in this session is listening. The therapist asks each family member to review his/her experience of the therapy from start to finish. The therapist may help this process along by demarcating the phases of the therapy and emphasizing certain issues that arose for each family member in the process. The process should begin with the parents, followed by the patient and siblings. Care should be taken to include all family members, though, by necessity, more time is likely to be taken up by the parents and the patient. The therapist must carefully time this session so that no more than about half of the allotted time is used for this reminiscence. Particular strategies that can be used include asking each family member to describe how things have changed in terms of BN and family functioning since treatment began. The more specific the examples the family members offer, the clearer it is to everyone just how much has changed. This procedure can also help family members identify areas of continued growth and those that need improvement.

Common Questions and Troubleshooting for Phase III

• *What if the family persists in using bulimic behaviors and food and weight concerns in the adolescent–parent communication?* It may be that in some families, even though the worst bulimic symptoms and related concerns have passed, there is a persistent pattern of using worries about binge eating and purging as a way of communicating with one another. In these cases, the therapist's aim should be to identify the reasons that this focus remains. For instance, parents are overly anxious that the illness has not been resolved, and they find it difficult to relate to their adolescent in any other way than through being worried about the eating disorder. In such cases, the therapist will reiterate a realistic appraisal of the adolescent's clinical status and through psychoeducation, try to reassure the parents that their daughter is indeed better. The therapist will direct conversation away from the illness and point out to the parents, in a very direct way, the actual topic of discussion. Such a discussion about adolescence may help to refocus the family on more appropriate concerns. At this juncture the therapist may find it helpful to directly explore the preoccupations with bulimic symptoms of the family as a whole to gain a better understanding of such a continued focus.

• *What if the parents deny that there are other adolescent issues or problems?* Some families find it difficult to admit that there may be problematic issues beyond BN present in their families. If such is the case, it is important that the therapist guide the parents and adolescent toward recognition of any problem areas identified by the therapist. It can be helpful to use the strategy of a general review that is provided in the therapeutic intervention described on pages 211–212 to discuss the typical issues associated with adolescents. This way, any problematic issue can be identified in a nonpathological manner and a discussion of the issue(s) can occur in a way that is noncritical of the family.

• *What if the parents are not involved in the review of the adolescent developmental process?* One possible problem associated with the therapeutic intervention of reviewing adolescent development is that the therapist can become a lecturer on adolescence. Consequently, the therapist might inadvertently create the scenario where she/he is doing most of the talking and the parents (and the adolescent, to some degree) are not directly involved in the review of these adolescent issues. Although the therapist should be seen as an expert guide in the area of the adolescent developmental process, this discussion should be a collaborative one with the family that provides opportunities for interaction. Should the therapist find him/herself in this position, he/she can shift to a focus on the parents' experience of their own adolescence as a way to solicit their participation in this discussion. It is helpful to directly ask the parents to revisit some of their own challenges when they were adolescents. It not only helps to make them a part of this discussion, it also may help the parents to revisit their own strategies in helping their daughter negotiate similar challenges, albeit 30 years later.

• *What if the parents do not see the value in spending time together as a couple, separate from their children, in order to nurture their marital relationship?* Rarely do partners believe that they do not need to spend any time together as a couple and apart from their children. However, in families where the patient is an only child, partners may be less willing to spend time apart from their child. In such cases, it is helpful to remind the parents that soon their daughter will be leaving home and that it may be good practice for them and for her to do things separately.

Conclusion of Phase III

In a relatively uncomplicated case of adolescent BN, the therapist should attempt to bring treatment of the BN to a close within about 20 sessions in a period of 6 months. If at this point there are still lingering issues that are not related to the eating disorder, such as an unresolved comorbid condition or specific adolescent developmental challenge, the therapist should make an appropriate referral for ongoing treatment. However, in our experience, a large majority of cases successfully terminate treatment within this specified time period. In the next chapter, we present a case in action that should demonstrate most of the strategies and challenges outlined in Chapter 12.

CHAPTER 13

Phase III in Action

In this chapter we provide an example of a session at the beginning of Phase III. It begins with a brief review of the progress made by the patient and her family, a reminder of the three phases of treatment, and that they are now embarking on the third and final phase of treatment. Because of the satisfactory progress demonstrated in treatment, the therapist starts out with a review of adolescent development and its relevance to the patient.

The major goals for this phase of treatment are:

- To establish that the adolescent–parent relationship is no longer defined by BN symptoms.
- To review adolescent issues with family and to model problem solving of these type of issues.
- To terminate treatment.

In order to accomplish these goals, the therapist should undertake the following interventions:

1. Review adolescent issues with family and model problem solving of these types of issues.
2. Involve parents in review of adolescent issues.
3. Ask parents how much they are doing as a couple, separate from their children.
4. Delineate and explore adolescent themes.
5. Prepare for challenges and issues that may arise in the future.
6. Terminate treatment.

Clinical Background

Beth is a 15-year-old Caucasian female presenting with a diagnosis of BN. Her height is 63 inches, and her weight is 127.8 pounds with a BMI of 22. Ideally, Beth would like to weigh 115 pounds. She lives with her parents outside the city. Her three brothers have all left home. Beth presented to the clinic with bulimic symptoms, 8 months in duration, characterized by twice-a-day binge eating followed by self-induced vomiting. No laxative, diuretic, or diet pill use was reported, but the occasional compensatory exercise rituals were present. Beth has regular menstrual cycles and is not taking oral contraceptives. She denied any functional impairment as a result of her eating disorder and did not present with other comorbidities.

Review Adolescent Issues with Family and Model Problem Solving of These Types of Issues

THERAPIST: So we have completed Phase I and Phase II and now we are moving into Phase III, as we talked about. Because your daughter had an eating disorder we focused all our time on that, which we had to do until we knew that she was no longer bothered by the binge eating or the purging. Because she has not had any binges or purges for the past couple of months now, we can address some of these other issues that we have put on the shelf, so to speak. Because your daughter is an adolescent, there is a whole host of other issues, as you probably know, that go on. It isn't just that you dealt with an eating disorder. You have raised three boys through adolescence, so you know what that is about, but with a girl there are many more issues that probably arise. I want to start by talking a little about the three distinct phases of adolescence, and then we are going to cover each of those stages of adolescence during the remainder of treatment. Part of this is understanding whether any specific issues have come up in each of these stages for Beth. (*turning to Beth*) And part of this is also understanding that your parents were once adolescents and what their (*laugh*) adolescence was like and how that compares with yours. So, bear with me with this little tutorial here. As I mentioned, we can think about adolescence as being composed of three different stages: There is the early stage of adolescence between the ages of 12 and 14, and that's really primarily associated with the physical changes of puberty. The next stage is the middle stage of adolescence, and that is typically from ages 14 to 16. Although we put ages on these stages, kids can move through them at different ages. Middle adolescence is concerned with peers taking on an increased importance in the adolescent's life and, Mom and Dad, you may feel a little bit like you have been put on the back burner, as her peers become really important. Part of this stage is also her developing thinking about sexuality as well as thinking about who it is she would like to date—those types of experiences. I see a little eye roll from Dad over there, so we'll have plenty to talk about right? (*laughing*)

The above overview (and its continuation below) of adolescence is an example of the type of concise description that a therapist can provide to orient families to possible additional issues. The particular structure has the advantage of being relatively straightforward, while offering clear developmental points the family can use to pinpoint their own concerns.

Involve Parents in Review of Adolescent Issues

FATHER: Yeah, we had an experience over the weekend.

THERAPIST: Yeah (*laughing*), so you know that is part and parcel of what the middle stage of adolescence is about. I think your daughter is right in the middle, between middle adolescence and later adolescence, which is typically 16–19 years of age, and is concerned with moving on into adulthood and being able to make independent decisions: going off to college, entering the work environment, and entering into longer-term interpersonal relationships—in short, how to successfully transition from being an adolescent to being a young adult. Like I said, we are going to talk about each stage in turn. I think it could be really helpful for you [the parents] to think about your own experiences, in addition to Beth's. I think in a lot of ways it's so great that we are at this point in treatment, and everyone in this room has done a wonderful job of helping Beth. Beth, you are getting better, and I know for myself as a therapist, it's so nice to talk about other things, knowing that these harmful symptoms are under control. It's an opportunity to take these issues that were on the shelf or on the back burner and move them more forward. They're issues that are very important, and the eating disorder unfortunately has a way of coming first and foremost in a lot of situations. The eating disorder makes the person who is going through adolescence not necessarily able to progress like someone without an eating disorder would progress. That said, maybe we should start off with the first stage, the early stage of adolescence, that is primarily concerned with puberty and the associated physical changes. (*turning to parents*) I mentioned how you have already been through adolescence with your three boys, but you know puberty affects girls and boys very differently, especially in our culture. Girls are expected to fit in or, if they are maturing too early through this stage, then it's thought of as if there is something not right; she's too young to be going through all of this or she's maturing too early. That's thought of as not normative, whereas boys, on the other hand, are different; they're expected to mature early and if they get taller and bigger, then that's acceptable. Girls, in contrast, are in some ways heavily judged in this culture on their physical appearance. Puberty can be a hard developmental stage, particularly for someone who has an eating disorder. So, I don't know if you are willing to talk about what that was like for you? You can talk about anything you are comfortable with, of course, particularly in relation to this stage when there are physical changes in your body and how you coped with those changes. Don't worry, you'll all get a chance to chime in (*all laugh*).

Although this may be somewhat of a monologue, the therapist covers essential ground in a related way, carefully reviewing the stages of adolescence and why this information is relevant for this family and their discussions at this stage of treatment. Although the therapist directed most of this discussion to the parents, and wanted them to start talking about their experiences during adolescence, it is Beth who answers first.

BETH: Badly.
THERAPIST: Yeah?
BETH: Um, that was when I started gaining weight, and that was when the most of the teasing went on.
THERAPIST: Teasing by whom, your peers or your . . . ?
BETH: Yeah, and my brothers somewhat.
THERAPIST: When you started to reach puberty, that is when you lost your weight?
BETH: No, I started my period in fifth grade.
THERAPIST: So you were . . .

BETH: I weighed 130 pounds in fifth grade, which is about what I weigh now.

THERAPIST: Okay.

BETH: So it was just really tough mostly because I wasn't used to having to watch my weight. Growing up with three brothers, you want to fit in with them first.

THERAPIST: Sure.

BETH: So you eat what they eat, and do what they do, and girls can't eat what guys can eat.

THERAPIST: Right.

BETH: So I had to figure that out, and my parents are some of those people who have you clean your plate.

THERAPIST: The Clean Plate Club?

BETH: I still haven't gotten past that; I can't *not* finish something. That was probably the toughest stage for me.

FATHER: When did you lose the weight?

BETH: The summer between seventh and eighth grade. 'Cause I went in to therapy the first time the winter of ninth grade.

FATHER: And that was because you had some episodes of not eating?

BETH: Mostly mom put me in therapy because I started having periods of not eating well.

FATHER: Were you . . . anorexic?

Father demonstrates remarkable lack of knowledge about the development of the eating disorder in his daughter. This was not perceived by the therapist as lack of interest or care on his part, but rather as reflective of the degree to which this family separated "women's issues" from "men's issues." However, Father is now becoming more acquainted with the history of his daughter's illness. Instead of talking about their own adolescence, the parents let their daughter explore her early stages of puberty and the development of her eating disorder.

BETH: No, the therapist said that I was fine . . . not anorexic . . . she said that falling under 100 pounds would be anorexic.

THERAPIST: You were teetering on the verge.

ALL: Yeah.

MOTHER: She was 101.

BETH: I was 105.

FATHER: She lost so much weight that her body wouldn't work.

THERAPIST: How did that come about? You mentioned that that was a hard stage for you because you ate what your brothers ate and then you started to realize . . .

BETH: I don't know, it happened really fast, just 1 month during the summer. I lost a lot. I must have lost 10 or 15 pounds in 1 month. I had already lost a little weight between fifth- and seventh-grade year, maybe 10 pounds or something, so I was down to about 120, and then that 1 month I got all the way down to like 105.

THERAPIST: Wow, through dieting or something else?

BETH: Yeah, something came over me, I could go for days without eating.

THERAPIST: (turning to her parents) Were you aware that this was going on?

FATHER: Yes, she was a stout, chubby girl, and she got teased about it all the time, relentlessly. It was a couple of kids in her class. Then she matured physically a little bit and started taking on the shape of a woman. She is a cute girl to start with, so some of the boys starting noticing her. Adolescent boys, well, they are not too bright.

THERAPIST: Yeah (laughing).

FATHER: We could imagine those boys thinking, "She doesn't look so bad after all." So as soon as she starts looking a little nice, well, they tease her even more for her attention.

THERAPIST: I see.

BETH: That's his theory . . .

FATHER: What?

BETH: That's your theory.

FATHER: Well, I mean, gosh, if there was a claim that . . . they wanted your attention so often and they were just . . .

BETH: Not before I lost all the weight.

FATHER: No, I mean, this was as you were losing more. The more weight you lost, the more they teased you about it. It shouldn't make any sense, but that's what happened.

BETH: No, they teased me the most about it in third through fifth grade, when I was at my heaviest.

FATHER: They still kept teasing you, though, when you started losing weight.

BETH: Yeah, but it didn't get worse.

FATHER: No. Well, maybe not, but they were teasing you for a different reason. The boys were older than her and they just wanted her attention.

MOTHER: Yeah, but the girls were worse than the boys sometimes.

THERAPIST: How so?

BETH: No, the boys were always worse. The girls never teased me that bad. I mean, there would be an occasional comment. When I started basketball in fifth grade, my nickname was "Butterball."

THERAPIST: Are you kidding?

BETH: No. I don't know how I got that nickname, but yeah.

FATHER: But when she first started losing a little weight and started physically maturing, like a woman, she was really happy about it. She got a lot of attention, and even a few of the mothers would say, "Yeah, boy, she's really shaping u" They would tell us about her, you know. But it seemed like one thing fed another. She liked the way she looked, she liked the attention, so she pushed it a little further.

BETH: Well, I don't think I really knew the balance of where I could stop dieting and what I could eat to keep myself like that. I didn't really know—I'm still struggling with it—but it's hard to find that balance of where I can stop. I was just so afraid of gaining it back that—heck, losing it is easier, you know. I guess I thought "I've already got this down, why not just keep doing it?"

THERAPIST: Right, and you were so afraid of gaining back the weight. It's not fun to be . . .

BETH: . . . the fat kid

THERAPIST: . . . the brunt of jokes, yeah. Well, that what's so hard about being an adolescent. Kids can be incredibly cruel and say things that you can't help but interpret as nasty or worse.

FATHER: I mean, this was so stupid. Here she was down to 110, and she even looked a little slender . . . to us, she started looking a little slender. . . . You know, we were okay with it. First we saw her walking with her head down. Then we heard the kids still being mean and we thought, "Oh, this is stupid." They just wanted her attention.

BETH: Well, it was down to where I could see my whole rib cage and my pelvic bones.

THERAPIST: Wow.

FATHER: Yeah, I remember that.

MOTHER: I mean the teasing went so far that I talked to a teacher I respected pretty much.

BETH: Yeah, bad idea.

MOTHER: I told her what was going on, and she told me that Beth had to grow thicker skin and that there was nothing they could do about it.

THERAPIST: Really? That's a shame.

BETH: With kids, if you yell at them, they will just do it more.

MOTHER: Sometimes going to an authority figure makes it worse, but I thought this was a situation that needed some addressing. You know, they were vicious. I would come home—it was right after I started working—and find her sobbing in the chair.

BETH: I don't remember crying that much.

MOTHER: You cried a lot.

BETH: No.

MOTHER: You did that a lot, Beth.

BETH: See, I remember crying maybe once or twice but never as much as they say.

MOTHER: But you would think, as much as she got teased, that they [teachers] would notice and be able to say *something*. We had a son who got bullied, and he said to us, "Please don't say anything because it only makes it worse."

BETH: Well, it does.

THERAPIST: What was your philosophy, Beth, at the time?

BETH: Well, if kids figure out that you are telling somebody about it, then they know it is getting to you and so they are just going to just do it more because they know they can get to you.

FATHER: With her losing weight, she picked up some energy—at least, we thought she had—and she got really athletic in basketball. She kind of became a leader on the team. She is very smart too, so now, not only did she look like she lost weight, she also looked nice, but she was a leader in the class too and that helped a little bit. The kids started looking up to you in basketball. After that you really got some confidence about you.

It is noteworthy perhaps that some of the triggering events related to the development of BN are discussed for the first time here. In other treatment types these might have been where treatment began. Examining these triggering events without the behaviors and thoughts of BN present changes the ability of both the adolescent and the parents to discuss them and think about their past and current import. It is also important to note the increased prompting of Beth during this session. The therapist would not allow the parents to talk about their adolescent without checking in with her to see whether she agreed or disagreed. The opinion of the adolescent will be increasingly sought as this treatment draws to a close.

THERAPIST: Is that true?

BETH: Yeah. I guess a little bit, I don't know.

THERAPIST: Insult can be a hard thing for anyone to hear.

FATHER: She couldn't walk down the hall without the boys trying to get her attention.

THERAPIST: So what your dad is talking about . . . had the teasing kind of crossed the threshold so that they were now doing it to get your attention because they liked you? It sounds like that is why you were saying those adolescent boys are not too bright or too swift for appreciating Beth.

BETH: (*laughing*) That is his theory, I don't know.

FATHER: I don't know . . . she just made this big change from being . . .

BETH: . . . short little fat kid.

FATHER: Well, okay, I wasn't going . . .

BETH: It was true.

FATHER: Then she started losing weight and she didn't know where to stop.

Delineate and Explore Adolescent Themes

Revisiting the time when Beth's eating disorder started seemed an important theme in terms of her adolescent development. Here, though, with the luxury of recovery, Beth and her family can carefully look at the origins of her eating disorder, almost dissecting it, but from a psychologically healthier position than at the start of treatment, and therefore they are much more likely to benefit from this kind of discussion.

THERAPIST: Why is that? That might be something good to talk about. You said it was hard to find that balance. And I am sure that you were talking about how you got a lot of attention or positive reinforcement . . .

BETH: Oh, yeah.

THERAPIST: . . . for losing weight. So it is hard. We all like to hear positive things about ourselves so we continue the things for which we are getting the positive attention.

BETH: And it's hard to see yourself as good enough. Even when I was at 105 pounds, I could always find fat somewhere that I wanted to get rid of.

THERAPIST: Yeah, it's a never-ending quest.

BETH: It *still* is now. I am still not satisfied with myself, but I don't think I ever will be. I've never had that much self-confidence (*laughing*).

MOTHER: There's always something too small or too big, you know? I don't think there is a woman who can say she is completely happy with the way she looks. Even the models—none of them would even say they are totally satisfied with how they look, because no woman is ever totally satisfied, I don't think, with how they look.

THERAPIST: Well, you raise a good point. The term has been coined "normative discontent," and it is this very thing. It's become normative in this culture, and other cultures, to never be completely satisfied with how one looks, and I think it's particularly exaggerated in females, although it even exists in males. I think there are magazines for males that never existed a while ago—*Men's Health*, for instance. You are supposed to look a certain way, but I think it's particularly hard for females. That's why this whole stage of early adolescence is about coming to terms with these physical changes that are happening to your body. You're supposed to look like an adolescent, as your dad talked about, a young woman with curves and all that.

BETH: Well, no, actually I started purging in April of my eighth-grade year. It wasn't long after I got out of treatment.

THERAPIST: This is treatment for anorexia, for losing too much weight?

BETH: Yeah, I think I started that summer. It wasn't that much, maybe once a month, and then it just progressed.

FATHER: You didn't look too bad to me and then you gained a few pounds back and I thought "Ah, she's fine." We're paying for that now.

THERAPIST: (*to the mother*) What do you think?

BETH: Yeah, what's your opinion of that treatment, Mom? Did you feel like it was necessary or if it was serious?

FATHER: I don't know, she's always . . .

BETH: Why don't you let her speak first?

MOTHER: I was always one who does what the doctors say, and if they say "you do it," I do it. He [the father] is always the one who says we don't really need to do it, we can do this and we will be fine. But she [Beth] was fighting it, she didn't like it.

BETH: I didn't like it at all.

MOTHER: She didn't like her therapist. She didn't want to go, and so we made an agreement that once she started her periods again, she could quit.

BETH: About 2 weeks or a month into it . . .

THERAPIST: You got your period back?

BETH: Yeah, so I said, "Okay, I am done with this."

THERAPIST: So getting your period was the saving grace, huh?

BETH: Yeah.

MOTHER: I was fighting her and fighting him [the father].

THERAPIST: And you didn't like that because you felt like you were in the middle of it?

MOTHER: Yeah.

BETH: One night after I had been in therapy for a week and had gained back 3 pounds, I just started balling.

THERAPIST: Really?

BETH: Just uncontrollably, and I said, "I don't want to do this any more! This sucks so bad! I'm going to get fat!" She wanted me to gain back, like, 10 pounds I think it was.

THERAPIST: That must have felt terrible?

MOTHER: Yes, she was scared.

BETH: I was scared out of my mind. (*laughing*)

THERAPIST: Because 10 pounds seemed like 100 pounds?

BETH: I thought, 10 pounds on top of what I weigh already is just insane and I just . . . ugggh . . . I fought it so bad.

FATHER: Well, her body had to be regular, so she had to gain a little something, do something, to function a little more.

BETH: It was bad because I already had all these clothes. I was wearing a size one.

THERAPIST: Wow.

BETH: Yeah and (*laughing*) . . . then as I gained weight, you know, I knew I needed a bigger size, but . . . you can't admit to yourself that you've gone up a size.

THERAPIST: You should be able to fit into them because you once fit into them. It's difficult having an illness that gets you to think that that's an appropriate size or that that's where your body is supposed to be, even though all the other signs point to it not being healthy.

MOTHER: And she had worked hard to get to where she was at, she just didn't want to give that up yet.

The therapist allows the adolescent and her family to explore the origins of her illness but continues to bring the discussion back to events surrounding the onset of BN.

THERAPIST: If we particularly think about the stage of adolescence you were in, of the physical changes, when the therapist said you needed to gain 10 pounds, what were some of your thoughts?

BETH: I was trying to prepare myself for high school, and nobody wants to go into high school as the fat kid because that just wouldn't work. I knew that. So I just...I had worked so hard to get where I was, I didn't want to give that up. Gaining weight made me feel like, "What did I do all this for? This is absolutely ridiculous."

MOTHER: But then you started the intense exercising. I mean, Dad and I would have to stop her because if she couldn't get outside [because of the weather] she would be on the stairs. She would be up the stairs, then all the way down to the basement, back up, back down, and you couldn't stop her. For a long time she would just run, run, run, up the stairs. And we would have to say "cool it." It's fine.

BETH: I would exercise for maybe an hour or 2 hours a night.

MOTHER: Oh, at least. Then she would go down to the basement and we would hear her doing jumping jacks. And then after we'd go to bed, we'd hear her upstairs doing more intense exercise. She may eat a little more, but then she tried to exercise it all off.

THERAPIST: I see. So it was a way of compensating.

MOTHER: Yeah.

THERAPIST: "If I have to eat, I'll exercise as much as possible to make sure that I don't gain weight."

MOTHER: Right, and we finally had to say "Slow down!"

FATHER: Well, exercising—hard exercising—produces something in the brain that—that when you—can't relax . . .

BETH: You get endorphins.

THERAPIST: They charge up your body.

FATHER: She was getting ticked off because I'd turn the lights off early. I like a nice, quiet daughter.

BETH: He likes everybody in bed by 9 o'clock.

FATHER: At 9 (*laughing*).

BETH: Don't even get me started.

FATHER: She was upstairs with the light on, and you could hear her running around up there, and it just . . . oh, man. I probably told her, "If you're going to exercise, you can exercise early in the evening so you can wind down for an hour or two, so you can go to bed."

BETH: And as an adolescent I said, "No, I'm going to exercise when I want to, and you can shove that in your peace pipe and smoke it."

FATHER: We were fighting the exercise thing when we started figuring out why the toilet wasn't working. It was because of the purging.

THERAPIST: So it sounds like you were attempting to regulate this body that has a mind of its own?

BETH: Yeah, it just won't cooperate.

THERAPIST: I'm assuming you both (*to parents*) were helpful in giving her some pearls of wisdom.

MOTHER: Well, we tried.

THERAPIST: What things did you try?

BETH: Well, whatever he said, I didn't do it.

THERAPIST: Is that right?

FATHER: No, we didn't know what to do with this stupid thing we had.

MOTHER: John would try to talk to her and she would just . . .

FATHER: When I would say something to her, we would just butt heads.

THERAPIST: Is this about the exercising?

BETH: About anything!

FATHER: She would take off on me like a lawnmower!

BETH: I just looked at him and I was like, "What could he know about exercising," about diet!

THERAPIST: It seemed a little hypocritical.

BETH: I just didn't understand how he knew what he was talking about.

FATHER: I went through 4 years of football and all that.

BETH: Yeah, but guys' metabolisms are much different than girls'.

FATHER: Well, I mean as far as gaining weight, losing weight, and getting in shape—I went through that.

BETH: For a guy.

THERAPIST: Well, that's interesting.

FATHER: It's an extreme.

With the discussion going somewhat astray, the therapist turns to the mother in an attempt to solicit her experiences around body shape and weight when she was an adolescent.

THERAPIST: That's interesting. You know, certainly there are eating disorders in athletes and problems with enhancing performance, and so men are certainly not immune, in particular, young men in sports and athletics. But we also have another female in this room, your mom, and she went through the same developmental stage. I wonder if you wouldn't mind sharing with Beth some of your own thoughts or your own feelings about going through the exact same thing she went through. I don't mean to be putting you on the spot. I really am not. Feel free to pass the hot potato if you'd like.

MOTHER: When I was growing up, until I graduated from high school, I never did have to fight my weight. But back then girls were accepted more as—I mean, I wore a size 11/12, and I was considered one of the thinner girls. It wasn't a size 5 like she tries to fit into, so . . .

BETH: Tries?! Thank you, Mom. (*laughing*)

MOTHER: It wasn't that thin, thin, thin thing back then. But after I got out of high school, I gained some weight. Before I met John, I lost some weight; otherwise he wouldn't have dated me because I thought I was fat. But once he saw that I'd lost weight, he got interested.

THERAPIST: Is that true?

MOTHER: Yeah, that's true, he told me that. (*laughing*)

FATHER: Yeah, I know.

MOTHER: He saw me at a football game.

FATHER: I saw her at a football game and . . .

MOTHER: And you thought I was a little bit too hefty.

FATHER: I ended up seeing her sister, who married my best friend, and they got married earlier so that's how we met. I saw her all along.

THERAPIST: That's right, at the wedding—I remember you talking about that before in one of our sessions.

FATHER: Yeah she came to one of our football games as a senior and . . .

MOTHER: I was a little bit hefty.

FATHER: A little bit, I thought. I really don't remember what I thought.

MOTHER: You told me one time.

FATHER: I think I did think she was a little more on the heavy side, but that's just, you know, I was just some stupid boy at that time. The first thing you look at, you think of sex you know. (*snickering*) I mean, you do, you know what I mean? Because like it or not . . .

BETH: But do we have to say it around . . . I'm going to stretch.

THERAPIST: You're just getting uncomfortable.

When the parents do start talking about their own adolescence and sexual awakenings, Beth gets very uncomfortable and wishes to be excused. The therapist sees this immediately and tries to be sympathetic to her concerns. The parents continue their discussion about dating, though.

FATHER: That's just what high school boys look at, I mean what the heck. They don't know.

MOTHER: I knew I did have a problem, like Beth did. I was teased a lot. I was teased a lot at school.

THERAPIST: Teased a lot for your weight or for other issues?

MOTHER: Not for my weight, no, for other things.

THERAPIST: Okay, so you know what that feels like or you can empathize with your daughter who's going through that.

MOTHER: Oh, there was one time I had to go hide in the bathroom when I was in seventh grade because they started calling me names when I went through the gym.

BETH: I don't know why they would.

MOTHER: Well, I was the geek.

THERAPIST: Studious.

MOTHER: Yeah, so then they started calling me . . .

THERAPIST: Well, being called a geek is a good thing in my book.

MOTHER: But they started calling me these things, so I just went down and hid in the bathroom and went out the other way. But I got teased some.

THERAPIST: Getting back to the teacher's comment of, "Oh, you just need to develop a thick skin." I know people say that, but that's easier said than done.

MOTHER: That's hard to do.

THERAPIST: In a lot of ways it would be tempting to say, "Well, then, they need to develop a thinner skin," or they need to develop more sensitivity.

MOTHER: I felt really bad when she came up with all these problems. I thought, well maybe if I had gone in and had been more adamant about things, maybe I didn't defend my child enough, you know.

BETH: It wouldn't have helped.

THERAPIST: You have those thoughts, but at least you think that that could have helped.

BETH: No, the teachers wouldn't have done anything and even if they had it just would have made it worse. The kids just would have been worse. So there was nothing you could do.

THERAPIST: You felt a little powerless, and I'm sure that John, you did as well.

FATHER: Absolutely. We had a son right before, in high school at the same time she was struggling with this anorexia, and he in his freshmen and sophomore years, in particular, he was picked on. We were actually getting worried that it might be getting out of hand, and we just said something to the principal.

MOTHER: Yeah, but we didn't do anything until he started coming home with bruises.

THERAPIST: Really?

FATHER: We just gritted out teeth and knew that time would take care of it. Then his junior year it started to subside and he was firmed up. He was fine his junior and senior years. The boy is tough to take care of.

MOTHER: I saw somebody go up and twist his ears off, and John had to hold me back. It's like, I want to go up there and just pull *his* ear off.

THERAPIST: Absolutely.

MOTHER: What right does he have to do that to my child? And it's the saddest thing . . .

BETH: Yeah, but if you do that . . . oh my gosh!

MOTHER: I know, I know.

BETH: You know what would happen.

MOTHER: But you know, as parents, you just want to go up there and do something for your kid.

FATHER: I always held her back.

THERAPIST: You talked about how you were concerned about both your son as well as Beth. You know you'd see the visible bruises on your son, which is very scary, but in many ways . . .

MOTHER: But we didn't see hers.

THERAPIST: Yeah, there are bruises on the inside. They're both very. . . . neither one is less traumatic than the other and they both leave scars and bruises and obviously.

FATHER: Our oldest son lived through high school. He was one of the leaders in his class and everything was good.

BETH: He was kind of a dork.

FATHER: What?

BETH: He was!

FATHER: He was, but he got away with it.

BETH: Yeah.

FATHER: He just got away with . . . everything worked for him. The second one, Jeremy, is where we noticed the trouble.

BETH: Jim [oldest son] had this thing, he was okay with not fitting in. I mean, he had his group of friends, like three or four friends, and they just all agreed that they were dorks (*laughing*). It was okay. But it's hard to find a group of friends that's okay with being dorks anymore.

FATHER: But then Jeremy . . .

BETH: . . . just wanted to fit in.

FATHER: He's very sensitive. We had a problem with a couple of teachers who said some very mean things, very stupid, and we still have trouble with the same teachers. The teachers, when he was on scholastic bowl, they said he wasn't smart enough. The teacher told him this, and we got some firsthand accounts of that.

THERAPIST: The teacher said this directly to him?

MOTHER: One teacher said, "Let's put Jeremy in," and the other teacher said, "I don't think he's really very bright," right in front of the other kids. That was the last scholastic bowl he ever went to. He tried the next year at the same school.

FATHER: The same thing happened three or four times, and he really got down on himself. When Joe came along, we thought, "Oh, what are we going to do with this one?" But we tried to always stay back from their lives.

Beth is making a general comment about her parents, and her father in particular, not being able to give their adolescent children more "space." Whereas these issues would have been difficult to discuss in the earlier part of treatment, with the eating disorder tangled up with the issue of parental supervision, the family now has the opportunity to look at this more in the context of a healthy challenge from a healthy daughter who is approaching her 16th birthday.

BETH: Ehhhhhh.

THERAPIST: You feel like they needed to not interfere so much, Beth?

BETH: Yeah, I think, I don't know. I think that going and talking like they did—I know my mom went and talked to Jim's coach 'cause he got teased during basketball and . . .

MOTHER: It was Dad.

BETH: Somebody did. That just makes things worse. I know when I become a parent I'm not going to understand that, I'm going to want to protect my kid, but you just have to understand that this is something that kids have to get through on their own. Saying something will just make it worse.

FATHER: It did help him a little bit. Like I said, the principal got a couple of the teachers together so they had . . .

BETH: Yeah, but after that, when the teachers weren't watching, it got worse.

FATHER: Well, it slowed down after a little bit, and then he got older and more mature and these two or three bullies who were picking on him just stopped.

THERAPIST: I think what we're hinting at is the next stage of adolescence which is, as I mentioned when we first started talking, heavily about peers and fitting in. It matters what they think more than it matters what your parents think, and you take on some of their values.

BETH: Of course.

THERAPIST: Speaking of someone who's between middle adolescence and later adolescence, what Beth is striving to say is that it does make a big difference what your peers think, and she's also saying, it's a very difficult thing being a parent. As you (*to the mother*) said, every time you saw these bullies say mean remarks to your daughter, you both were just "I'd like to sock him," or I'd like to tell him where to stick it, or whatever you want to say.

FATHER: The middle stage of adolescence is painful to watch. That's the worst. Because you see your child making stupid decisions just to go along with the pack, and you can see it. It's very obvious. It's not hard to see.

BETH: I'm wondering if you both can remember back to your own middle adolescence . . .

MOTHER: Oh, sure.

FATHER: That might even make it worse! You could sure see it. But, Beth, thankfully, in the last few months we see a good decision, once in a great while, about everything.

THERAPIST: Just once in a great while?

FATHER: Well, she makes some stupid decisions.

MOTHER: It's hard to try to fit in. You know, it really is.

THERAPIST: Absolutely.

BETH: Especially in a town like Winnetka, where all these kids grew up, went to kindergarten together; they've been together forever. I've been with them for only 4 years and trying to fit in and become like they are . . .

THERAPIST: I see.

BETH: When they've been together for that long, it's just practically impossible.

THERAPIST: Your desire to fit in and conform is completely understandable.

You have, on top of a normal adolescent need to conform and fit in, there's this hurdle that they have all this history together. You must have thought, "I have to really back track here and make up for lost time."

FATHER: And Winnetka is really a . . .

BETH: They're stuck up.

MOTHER: It's a snooty town.

THERAPIST: Is that right?

ALL: Yeah.

THERAPIST: I have to remind myself to note that down: Never to travel to Winnetka.

MOTHER: It's okay, if you think of their town as the greatest, if you live in it. But going into it is hard.

FATHER: It's okay, they're just . . .

THERAPIST: . . . a close-knit group.

MOTHER: Yeah.

THERAPIST: And high school and adolescence are already cliquey enough.

MOTHER: Right.

FATHER: I think it's good that the kids went to a different grade school. I've said this several times: It will be painful for them to go to a new high school, but they'll be a leg up in college because they're used to all that change.

MOTHER: It does make it a little bit easier on them when they go to college, because they've already tried to fit in one place.

BETH: I couldn't imagine, oh my gosh, going to school with the same kids until college and then moving out the door.

THERAPIST: Yeah, so that's a silver lining, looking at it.

BETH: I don't really see it right now, though.

MOTHER: It's hard to see it now, though.

THERAPIST: More of a gray lining as opposed to a silver lining.

THERAPIST: College is an exciting thing to look forward to, if you can just get through this middle stage of adolescence.

FATHER: With peers she puts on such a stinking fuss. This one night she went out and came home and just bawled and whined to us about how important it was to do what her friends said, like, take the car and drop her off a little up the road. I mean, it was just stupid, but she just threw such a fit.

THERAPIST: Do you remember that night?

BETH: Oh, very clearly.

THERAPIST: Do you remember your dad and mom being irritated?

BETH: Yeah. And I understand where they're coming from, but it's still so hard to fit in, and in Winnetka there's nothing to do. There's Subway and McDonald's and that's about it.

THERAPIST: Well, that becomes very difficult for you guys, as parents. We talked a little bit about what it's like to be a female in this culture and get through adolescence with minimal scars. I think it is very difficult in this day and age to be an adolescent, pardon the pun, but it can be a nasty cocktail out there. Parents somehow supplying their children with alcohol and kids drinking as they'd want to fit in. It would be very difficult, I would imagine, for both of you to know . . .

FATHER: It was horrible.

THERAPIST: Where you're going to lay the law down or . . .

FATHER: We had our second son, who just wanted to live out there, and we just said, whatever.

THERAPIST: Yeah.

FATHER: When you have a 16- or 17-year-old child who absolutely refuses to do what you want him to and insists on having his own way, and he's strong-willed enough, there isn't a whole lot you can do about it.

THERAPIST: Right.

FATHER: You can't harm him physically or restrain him even if you wanted to—he's as big as we are, you can't do that. You don't have any options. We would get to the point—man, *I* would get to the point— where I wanted to kick him out of the house all the time and didn't know what to do. Beth comes along a little bit later and she breaks a few rules too, but she's not as bad. She's turned on me, but she's not so bad.

THERAPIST: That's high praise, it sounds like, from Dad.

BETH: Umm-hmm.

In this session early in Phase III the therapist is pleased with the ability of the parents to call upon their prior experiences—their own adolescence as well as their experience parenting their adolescent sons. The general themes that will be the subject of this phase are hinted at, particularly in the last set of exchanges. Although the patient's older brothers are no longer at home, it is possible the therapist might ask one or more of them to attend a session, if they can, to participate in this stage of treatment, because they might be able to share some of their challenges when they were adolescents. As mentioned before, not all points get addressed in a typical session.

Bring Session to a Close

As is the case with all sessions, the therapist makes a closing statement, albeit briefly in this instance.

> "Well, these are all issues that we're going to continue to talk about in the remainder of sessions, so we'll jump around from different stages, and just because we leave one stage for the next session doesn't mean we can't return back to it. Thanks for talking about things so candidly and openly, and I look forward to seeing you again in 3 weeks."

In this final phase of treatment, discussions about the eating disorder are not central to the sessions. The discussions will mostly center on adolescent development and the ways in which the adolescent will go forward in life, negotiating challenges, mostly on her own, but also with the help of her family when and if needed or appropriate. In the final chapter we provide a case study that takes the reader through an account of all three phases in the successful treatment of an adolescent with BN.

CHAPTER 14

Summary of a Completed Case

The case presented in this final chapter demonstrates how the family's help can be solicited, along with the collaboration of the adolescent, in restoring the adolescent's eating to healthy patterns once more. The treatment for this case was relatively uncomplicated and for the most part went according to plan. Jane, as we refer to the adolescent patient, was 17 years old at the time of presentation. She was a relatively well-adjusted young woman who had already made strides to establish her own identity and independence from her family. Indeed, her independence posed the unique challenge of engaging a young adult in a treatment that requires her parents to, at the very least, assist her in her efforts at recovery. The case of Jane demonstrates this delicate therapeutic "dance" very well and shows how the therapist succeeded in enlisting the help of Jane and both her parents in order to work as a team to bring about her recovery.

Presenting Problem

Jane, the younger of two daughters from an intact, two-parent home, is a 17-year-old with a 4-year history of an eating disorder. She reported a history of being overweight as a child and preteen. At the age of 13, weighing 200 pounds, she began dieting restrictively and lost over 100 pounds (reporting a weight of 95 pounds). From ages 13–15 her weight remained

---

A version of this case was first published in Le Grange, Lock, and Dymek (2003). Copyright 2003 by the Association of the Advancement of Psychotherapy. Adapted by permission.

stable at 95 pounds; she had amenorrhea, and she met diagnostic criteria for AN. At age 15, she started binge eating and purging through self-induced vomiting. Jane's mother called our clinic to set up an appointment for the initial assessment. The patient presented with a weight of 126.7 pounds at 5'5" (BMI = 21.1) and reported four binge-eating episodes per week, with self-induced vomiting, on average, twice per day. On examination, she also met criteria for a current major mood disorder as well as panic disorder. Both Jane and her parents were somewhat reluctant to engage in family treatment and requested individual therapy. However, Jane was randomly allocated to family treatment, and she and her parents entered a course of 20 manualized FBT sessions over a 6-month period. Most family sessions were conducted with Jane and her two parents. Two of the sessions were also conducted with her older sister, a college student, while she was home on breaks. The family declined any treatment for the comorbid disorders, claiming that prior psychotropic medications were "unhelpful."

Case Formulation

Although Jane's parents were concerned about her binge eating and purging, they nevertheless were anxious not to "overstep" their perceived limits on parental involvement given their daughter's age. The parents' hands-off approach to parenting, as well as Jane's semi-independence in most aspects of her late adolescent life, posed a potential challenge for a family-based approach. The parents' relationship and their past history of dealing with Jane's difficulties remained unclear, especially in terms of how well they would be able to work together as a united team in assisting Jane in overcoming her BN. From a practical standpoint, the parents' very separate career paths and time commitments to their employers posed an additional quandary about the feasibility of family treatment. The initial goal of treatment was to meet with all family members living in the same household in order to make an assessment of the patient and her family. Jane's older sibling was away at college and therefore did not participate in treatment, other than at times when she was home with her family during school breaks. More specifically, the goal this early on was to help the parents work out a way to assist Jane with her eating so as to begin the process of reestablishing healthy eating patterns.

Course of Treatment

One of the therapist's initial tasks is to begin the process of defining and enhancing parental authority around management of the eating disorder. Unlike with adolescent AN, this authority is diffused and takes on more of a collaborative quality because many adolescents with BN seem more independent than their counterparts with AN. The parents assist the adolescent with her eating, making sure healthy portions of food are consumed at regular and appropriate intervals and working out ways to prevent binge eating and purging. To achieve this goal, it is important for both parents to start the process of reestablishing healthy eating patterns as a united team in order to be effective in addressing the eating disorder symptoms. In addition to assessing the eating disorder, the purpose of the initial session is also to educate the family in terms of the nature and severity of the eating disorder, especially the secretiveness and shame that are associated with binge eating and purging. The therapist will argue that because adolescents are embedded in their families, it is often most helpful to have the parents on board as a primary resource in overcoming the BN. In the first session, Jane's parents questioned taking control over their daughter's eating, citing her age and the amount of time she spent away from home (e.g., at school, at band practice). However, her parents were sufficiently mobilized by the potential dangers of the disorder, and they agreed to move forward, as suggested by the therapist. Although Jane expressed some anxiety about parental involvement, she also expressed relief that she would have help with some of these decisions around food that had been so difficult for her. The therapist also made it clear to Jane that the treatment is indeed very respectful of her in that the parents' task is to help her overcome the eating disorder so that she can negotiate adolescence and young adulthood unencumbered by it. The therapist also took this stance to raise parental anxiety about the seriousness of the illness and externalized the illness in order to mobilize the parents to take charge of it. The first session was brought to closure with the request that the family return the following week with a picnic lunch that should include a dessert (or any food item typically on the patient's list of forbidden food that often serves as a binge trigger).

The main goal of the second session, the family meal, was to continue the process of assessment by observing the family while eating, so that the therapist could learn more about Jane's struggle to eat healthy portions. The family brought submarine sandwiches, chips, and soft drinks for their meal. For much of the session, they watched Jane pick at her meal and consume very little. The therapist assisted the parents in determining the amount of food that would be healthy for an adolescent female, and encouraged the parents to help Jane eat appropriate portions of the sandwich and a small portion of potato chips, which was on Jane's list of forbidden foods. The therapist's task was to help Jane verbalize her thoughts and feelings around having eaten "too much" or having eaten the "wrong foods" and to help the parents understand her struggle not to purge as she feels rising anxiety and guilt for having consumed the chips. The parents' task, in turn, was to appreciate how difficult this may be for Jane, to understand her guilt and shame around these behaviors, and to assist her in *not* purging by spending time with her post meal.

In reviewing the family's patterns around eating, it was learned that Jane's mother did most of the shopping and preparing of meals. However, the family rarely ate meals together because of their conflicting schedules. Jane was initially resistant to eating breakfast, complaining that "It makes me nauseous," and frequently eluded eating dinner with her mother, saying that she had already eaten. The parents were encouraged to find a way to work together to overcome these obstacles and ensure that Jane was receiving adequate nutrition at regular intervals. Despite Jane's initial reluctance and the time obstacles, her parents were quickly able to help her establish regular eating patterns. The therapist provided considerable encouragement of the family's attempts, and by the fourth session Jane was regularly eating three healthy meals per day. The remainder of the first phase of treatment was spent carefully reviewing with Jane and her parents what efforts they had made during the past week to make sure that Jane not only consumed three healthy meals per day, but also avoided binge eating or purging. Spending time with her, "supervising" her post meal, though, was only partially successful. As expected, Jane reported that she found her parents' watchful eyes helpful, but that their surveillance curtailed only some of the purging episodes. At other times when she felt upset and her parents were not around, she would purge, recognizing that this purging was more an attempt to deal with distressing feelings than actual concern about weight gain. Because Jane's eating was quickly normalized, the remainder of Phase I was spent assisting the parents in helping Jane find healthier alternatives to managing her emotions and thereby reduce purging. By the seventh session, Jane's purging was reduced to one time per week.

Phase II of treatment was approached when Jane's eating behaviors returned to a healthy pattern and her purging was much reduced. At this time, the therapist's task was to guide the parents to withdraw their direct involvement in Jane's meal decisions and to allow her eating to reflect the independence she had acquired in most other areas of her life. With her parents present, the issue of managing feelings through purging remained a central area of discussion, and the parents assisted Jane in working on difficult situations or feelings through healthy means as opposed to purging behaviors. For example, Jane frequently became very upset over different interpersonal situations and found herself purging to "numb" herself to the distress. The therapist encouraged Jane's parents to discuss such situations with her when they arose and to assist her in finding healthier solutions. Several sessions were also spent assisting Jane's parents in helping her develop a list of adaptive/coping behaviors in which she could engage to help manage her distress.

By the time Jane and her family approached the third and final phase of treatment, she was both binge and purge free. The remaining focus of treatment was a review of remaining adolescent developmental tasks with the patient and her family. The developmental tasks that Jane would have to negotiate in the near future were identified and the extent to which it would be appropriate for her parents to be involved with these tasks was explored. The main issues discussed were helping Jane develop appropriate boundaries with friends, her new boyfriend, and her parents. The therapist also facilitated family discussions about smoking, sex and birth control, and going away to college.

Treatment was concluded on a positive note with Jane symptom free and optimistic about her budding independence. In addition, Jane also noted that much of her depression and anxiety had dissipated over the course of treatment.

Outcome in Terms of Eating Disorder Symptomatology

Jane's subjective binge eating ceased early in treatment, and she reported no further episodes after the fourth treatment session. Although purging behavior continued somewhat longer, no further purging was reported after the 14th treatment session. At the end of FBT Jane was binge and purge free and reported that she was "beginning to eat like a normal person." She gained a few pounds during the initial sessions of treatment, but her weight soon stabilized in a healthy range, which she maintained throughout the last 6 months of treatment (BMI at time of termination was 22.9).

Clinical Issues and Summary

Despite its prevalence, BN in adolescents has received relatively little attention in the literature. Even though the systematic evaluation of effective treatments has just passed the first hurdle, in that two large randomized trials have now been completed, our knowledge of the clinical presentation of BN in this population is in its infancy. In this book we argued that a manualized FBT with proven efficacy for adolescent AN can similarly benefit adolescents with BN. We provided a rationale for FBT of BN and described the outline of this treatment approach. Albeit tentative at this stage, but similar to our FBT of AN, we found that a manualized version of FBT for BN can provide a consistent, focused, and directed intervention in both a clinical and research environment. In the development of this treatment manual we followed the following stages:

1. Reviewed the existing descriptions of family treatment for BN.
2. Reviewed the literature comparing adolescent AN and BN.
3. Reviewed and adapted our AN manual, given the former steps.
4. Piloted this revised manual with several cases prior to its implementation in a controlled treatment study.
5. Successfully implemented this manual in a recently completed randomized clinical trial at the University of Chicago (Le Grange, Rathauz, Crosby, & Leventhal, 2006).

At this relatively early stage of our work with the families of adolescents with BN, it is quite clear that the parental involvement in BN should be somewhat different from that for AN. BN poses a unique challenge to the adolescent and her parents, and greater flexibility around addressing the eating disorder symptoms is necessary. This, in addition to other significant differences between these two eating disorders, such as secrecy and shame in BN versus resilience and even pride in AN, as well as the notion that most adolescents with BN are developmentally on track whereas most adolescents with AN have fallen behind, have all been accommodated in the manualized treatment described in this clinician's manual. It is clear, though, that this new treatment has promise in alleviating bulimic symptoms in adolescents and that parents can be a helpful resource in therapy.

Conclusions

In summary, family therapy for adolescent BN might enable recovery without protracted outpatient treatment or hospital admission. Successful restoration of an adolescent's health, through a return to healthy eating habits and the absence of binge eating and purging, depends in large part on the parents' ability to assist their child in much the same way as do the parents of an adolescent with AN. However, more controlled treatment studies are required to further evaluate the efficacy of this treatment, which could enable us to comment more definitively about the role of the parents in the recovery from BN.

References

Ackard, D. M., Neumark-Sztainer, D., Hannan, P. J., French, S., & Story, M. (2001). Binge and purge behavior among adolescents: Associations with sexual and physical abuse in a nationally representative sample: The Commonwealth Fund survey. *Child Abuse and Neglect, 25*(6), 771–785.

Agras, W. S., & Kraemer, H. C. (1983). The treatment of anorexia nervosa: Do different treatments have different outcomes? *Psychiatric Annals, 13*, 928–935.

American Psychiatric Association. (1994). *Diagnostic and statistical manual of mental disorders* (4th ed.). Washington, DC: Author.

Attie, I., & Brooks-Gunn, J. (1989). Development of eating problems in adolescent girls: A longitudinal study. *Developmental Psychology, 25*, 70–79.

Bachrach, L. K., Guido, I. R., & Katzman, D. K. (1990). Decreased bone density in adolescent girls with anorexia nervosa. *Pediatrics, 86*, 440–447.

Baran, S. A., Weftzer, T. E., & Kaye, W. H. (1995). Low discharge weight and outcome in anorexia nervosa. *American Journal of Psychiatry, 152*(7), 1070–1072.

Bliss, E. L., & Branch, C. H. (1960). *Anorexia nervosa: Its psychology and biology.* New York: Hoeber.

Bossert, S. (1988). Modifications and problems of behavioral inpatient management of anorexia nervosa: A patient-suited approach. *Acta Psychiatrica Scandinavica, 77*(1), 105–110.

Bruch, H. (1973). *Eating disorders, obesity, anorexia nervosa, and the person within.* New York: Basic Books.

Bruch, H. (1995). *Conversations with anorexics.* New York: Basic Books.

Bryant-Waugh, R. J., Cooper, P. J., Taylor, C. L., & Lask, B. D. (1996). The use of the eating disorder examination with children: A pilot investigation. *International Journal of Eating Disorders, 19*, 391–397.

Burck, C., & Daniel, G. (1990). Feminism and strategic therapy: Contradiction or complementarity? In R. J. Perelberg & A. C. Miller (Eds.), *Gender and power in families* (pp. 82–103). London: Draper Campbell.

Casper, R. C., Hedeker, D., & McClough, J. F. (1992). Personality dimensions in eating disorders and their relevance for subtyping. *Journal of the American Academy of Child and Adolescent Psychiatry, 31*(5), 830–840.

Channon, S., De Silva, P., Hemsley, D., & Perkins, R. (1989). A controlled trial of cognitive-behavioral and behavioral treatment of anorexia nervosa. *Behaviour Research and Therapy, 27*(5), 529–535.

Childress, A. C., Brewerton, T. D., Hodges, E. L., & Jarrell, M. P. (1993). The Kids' Eating Disorder Survey (KEDS): A study of middle school students. *Journal of the American Academy of Child and Adolescent Psychiatry, 32*, 843–850.

Cloninger, C. R. (1986). A unified biosocial theory of personality and its role in the development of anxiety states. *Psychiatric Developments, 3*, 167–226.

Cloninger, C. R. (1987). A systematic method for clinical description and classification of personality variants. *Archives of General Psychiatry, 44*, 573–588.

Cloninger, C. R. (1988). A unified theory of personality and its role in the development of anxiety states: Reply to commentaries. *Psychiatric Developments, 6*, 83–120.

Cooper, Z., & Fairburn, C. (1987). The Eating Disorder Examination: A semi-structured interview for the assessment of the specific psychopathology of eating disorders. *International Journal of Eating Disorders, 6*, 1–8.

Crisp, A. H. (1985). Gastrointestinal disturbance in anorexia nervosa. *Postgraduate Medical Journal, 61*, 3–5.

Crisp, A. H. (1997). Anorexia nervosa as a flight from growth: Assessment and treatment based on the model. In D. M. Garner & P. E. Garfinkel (Eds.), *Handbook of treatment for eating disorders* (2nd ed., pp. 248–277). New York: Guilford Press.

Crisp, A. H., Hsu, L. K. G., Harding, B., & Hartshorn, J. (1980). Clinical features of anorexia nervosa: A study of 102 cases. *Journal of Psychosomatic Research, 24*, 179–196.

Crisp, A. H., Norton, K., Gowers, S., Hale, K. C., Boyer, C., Yeldham, D., et al. (1991). A controlled study of the effect of therapies aimed at adolescent and family psychopathology in anorexia nervosa. *British Journal of Psychiatry, 159*, 325–333.

Crowther, J. H., & Chernyk, B. (1986). Bulimia and binge eating in adolescent females: A comparison. *Addictive Behaviors, 11*(4), 415–424.

Crowther, J. H., Post, G., & Zaynor, L. (1985). The presence of bulimia in high schools. *Adolescence, 20*, 45–51.

Dare, C. (1985). The family therapy of anorexia nervosa. *Journal of Psychiatric Research, 19*(2–3), 435–443.

Dare, C., & Eisler, I. (1997). Family therapy for anorexia nervosa. In D. M. Garner & P. E. Garfinkel (Eds.), *Handbook of treatment for eating disorders* (2nd ed., pp. 307–324). New York: Guilford Press.

Dare, C., Eisler, I., Russell, G. F. M., & Szmukler, G. (1990). Family therapy for anorexia nervosa: Implications from the results of a controlled trail of family and individual therapy. *Journal of Marital and Family Therapy, 16*, 39–57.

Dare, C., Le Grange, D., Eisler, I., & Rutherford, J. (1994). Redefining the psychosomatic family: Family process of 26 eating disorder families. *International Journal of Eating Disorders, 16*, 211–226.

Dodge, E., Hodes, M., Eisler, I., & Dare, C. (1995). Family therapy for bulimia nervosa in adolescents: An exploratory study. *Special Issue: Eating Disorders, Journal of Family Therapy, 17*(1), 59–77.

Dolan, R. J., & Mitchell, J. A. (1988). Structural brain changes in patients with anorexia nervosa. *Psychiatric Medicine, 18*, 349–353.

Eckert, E. D., Halmi, K. A., Marichi, P., Grove, W., & Crosby, R. (1995). Ten-year follow up of anorexia nervosa: Clinical course and outcome. *Psychological Medicine*, 25(1), 143–156.

Eisler, I., Dare, C., Hodes, M., Russell, G. F. M., Dodge, E., & Le Grange, D. (2000). Family therapy for adolescent anorexia nervosa: The results of a controlled comparison of two family interventions. *Journal of Child Psychology and Psychiatry*, 41(6), 727–736.

Eisler, I., Dare, C., Russell, G. F. M., Szmukler, G., Le Grange, D., & Dodge, E. (1997). Family and individual therapy in anorexia nervosa: A 5-year follow-up. *Archives of General Psychiatry*, 54(11), 1025–1030.

Fabian, L., & Thompson, J. K. (1989). Body image and eating disturbances in young females. *International Journal of Eating Disorders*, 8, 63–74.

Fairburn, C. G., & Cooper, Z. (2003). Relapse in bulimia nervosa: Comment. *Archives of General Psychiatry*, 60(8), 850.

Fairburn, C. G., Cooper, Z., Doll, H. A., Norman, P., & O'Connor, M. (2000). The natural course of bulimia nervosa and binge eating disorder in young women. *Archives of General Psychiatry*, 57(7), 659–665.

Fairburn, C. G., Shafran, R., & Cooper, Z. (1999) A cognitive behavioral theory of anorexia nervosa. *Behaviour Research and Therapy*, 37, 1–13

Fichter, M., & Quadflieg, N. (2004). Twelve-year course and outcome of bulimia nervosa. *Psychological Medicine*, 34(8), 1395–1406.

Fisher, M., Golden, N. H., Katzman, D. K., Kreipe, R. E., Rees, J., Schebendach, J., et al. (1995). Eating disorders in adolescents: A background paper. *Journal of Adolescent Health*, 16, 420–437.

Franko, D. L., Keel, P. K., Dorer, D. J., Blais, M. A., Delinsky, S. S., Eddy, K. T., et al. (2004). What predicts suicide attempts in women with eating disorders? *Psychological Medicine*, 34(5), 843–853.

French, S. A., Story, M., Neumark-Sztainer, D., Downes, B., Resnick, M., & Blum, R. (1997). Ethnic differences in psychosocial and health behavior correlates of dieting, purging, and binge eating in a population-based sample of adolescent females. *International Journal of Eating Disorders*, 22(3), 315–322.

Garfinkel, P. E., & Garner, D. M. (1982). *Anorexia nervosa: A multidimensional perspective*. New York: Brunner/Mazel.

Garfinkel, P. E., & Garner, D. M. (Eds.). (1987). *The role of drug treatment for eating disorders*. New York: Brunner/Mazel.

Garner, D. M. (1993). Pathogenesis of anorexia nervosa. *The Lancet*, 341, 1632–1634.

Gillberg, I. C., Rastam, M., & Gillberg, L. (1994). Anorexia nervosa outcome: Six-years controlled longitudinal study of 51 cases including a population cohort. *Journal of the American Academy of Child and Adolescent Psychiatry*, 33(5), 729–739.

Golden, N. H., & Shenker, I. R. (1992). Amenorrhea in anorexia nervosa: Etiology and implications. *Adolescent Medicine: State of the Art Reviews*, 3, 503–517.

Golden, N. M., Kreitzer, P., & Jacobson, M. S., Chasalow, F. I., Schebendach, J., Freedman, S. M., et al. (1994). Disturbances in growth hormone secretion and action in adolescents with anorexia nervosa. *Journal of Pediatrics*, 125, 655–660.

Gowers, S., Norton, K., Halek, C., & Crisp, A. H. (1994). Outcome of outpatient psychotherapy in a random allocation treatment study of anorexia nervosa. *International Journal of Eating Disorders*, 15(2), 165–177.

Gull, W. W. (1874). Anorexia nervosa (apepsia hysterica, anorexia hysterica). *Transactions of the Clinical Society of London*, 7, 222–228.

Gwirtzman, H. E., Guze, B. H., & Yager, J. (1990). Fluoxetine treatment of anorexia nervosa: An open clinical trial. *Journal of Clinical Psychiatry*, 51, 378–382.

Haley, J. (1973). *Uncommon therapy: The psychiatric techniques of Milton H. Erickson.* New York: Norton.

Hall, A., & Crisp, A. H. (1987). Brief psychotherapy in the treatment of anorexia nervosa: Outcome at one year. *British Journal of Psychiatry*, 151, 185–191.

Harper, G. (1983). Varieties of failure in anorexia nervosa: Protection and parentectomy revisited. *Journal of the American Academy of Child Psychiatry*, 22, 134–139.

Herpertz-Dalmann, B. M., Wewetzer, C., Schulz, E., & Remschmidt, H. (1996). Course and outcome in adolescent anorexia nervosa. *International Journal of Eating Disorders*, 19(4), 335–345.

Herzog, D. B., Dorer, D. J., Keel, P. K., Selwyn, S. E., Ekeblad, E. R., Flores, A. T., et al. (1999). Recovery and relapse in anorexia and bulimia nervosa: A 7.5-year followup study. *Journal of the American Academy of Child and Adolescent Psychiatry*, 38(7), 829–837.

Herzog, D. B., Field, A. E., Keller, M. B., West, J. C., Robbins, W. M., Staley, B. A., et al. (1996). Subtyping eating disorders: Is it justified? *Journal of the American Academy of Child and Adolescent Psychiatry*, 37(7), 928–936.

Herzog, D. B., Greenwood, D. N., Dorer, D. J., Flores, A. T., Ekeblad, E. R., Richards, A., et al. (2000). Mortality in eating disorders: A descriptive study. *International Journal of Eating Disorders*, 28(1), 20–26.

Herzog, D. B., Keller, M. B., & Lavori, P. W. (1992). The prevalence of personality disorders in 210 women with eating disorders. *Journal of Clinical Psychiatry*, 53, 147.

Herzog, D. B., Sacks, N., Keller, M., Lavori, P., von Ranson, K., & Gray, H. (1993). Patterns and predictors of recovery in anorexia nervosa and bulimia nervosa. *Journal of the American Academy of Child and Adolescent Psychiatry*, 32(4), 835–842.

Hill, A. J., Weaver, C., & Blundell, J. E. (1990). Dieting concerns of 10-year-old girls and their mothers. *British Journal of Clinical Psychology*, 29, 346–348.

Hoberman, H. M., & Garfinkel, B. D. (1990). Completed suicide in children and adolescents: Erratum. *Journal of the American Academy of Child and Adolescent Psychiatry*, 29(1), 156.

Hodes, M., & Le Grange, D. (1993). Expressed emotion in the investigation of eating disorders: A review. *International Journal of Eating Disorders*, 13, 279–288.

Hoste, R., & Le Grange, D. (2006, June). *Expressed emotion among Caucasian and minority families of bulimic adolescents.* Paper presented at the International Conference of the Academy for Eating Disorders, Barcelona, Spain.

Howard, W., Evans, K., Quintero-Howard, C., Bowers, W., & Anderson, A. (1999). Predictors of success or failure of transition to day hospital treatment for inpatients with anorexia nervosa. *American Journal of Psychiatry*, 156, 1697–1702.

Hsu, L. K. G. (1986). The treatment of anorexia nervosa. *American Journal of Psychiatry*, 143, 573–581.

Hsu, L. K. G. (1990). *Eating disorders.* New York: Guilford Press.

Jager, B., Liedtke, R., Lamprecht, F., & Freyberger, H. (2004). Social and health adjustment of bulimic women 7–9 years following therapy. *Acta Psychiatrica Scandinavica*, 110(2), 138–145.

Jenkins, M. E. (1987). An outcome study of anorexia nervosa in an adolescent unit. *Journal of Adolescence*, 10(1), 71–81.

Jones, J., Bennett, S., Olmsted, M. P., Lawson, M. L., & Rodin, G. (2001). Disordered eating attitudes and behaviors in teenaged girls: A school-based study. *Canadian Medical Association Journal*, 165, 547– 552.

Jones, L. M., Halford, W. K., & Dooley, R. T. (1993). Long-term outcome of anorexia nervosa. *Behavior Change*, 10(2), 93–102.

Keel, P. K., Mitchell, J. E., Miller, K. B., Davis, T. L., & Crow, S. J. (2000). Social adjustment over 10 years following diagnosis with bulimia nervosa. *International Journal of Eating Disorders*, 27(1), 21–28.

Kennedy, S. H., & Garfinkel, P. E. (1989). Patients admitted to hospital with anorexia nervosa and bulimia nervosa: Psychotherapy, weight gain, and attitudes toward treatment. *International Journal of Eating Disorders*, 8(2), 181–190.

Kent, A., Lacey, H., & McClusky, S. E. (1992). Pre-menarchal bulimia nervosa. *Journal of Psychosomatic Research*, 36, 205–210.

Killen, J. D., Hayward, C., & Litt, I., (1992). Is puberty a risk factor for eating disorders? *American Journal of Diseases of Children*, 146, 323–325.

Killen, J. D., Taylor, C. B., Telch, M. J., Robinson, T. N., Maron, D. J., & Saylor, K E. (1987). Depressive symptoms and substance use among adolescent binge eaters and purgers: A defined population study. *American Journal of Public Health*, 77, 1539–1541.

Killen, J. D., Taylor, C. B., Telch, M. J., Saylor, K. E., Maron, D. J., & Robinson, T. N. (1987). Evidence for an alcohol stress link among normal weight adolescents reporting purging behavior. *International Journal of Eating Disorders*, 6(3), 349–356.

Kreipe, R. E. (1989). Short stature in females with anorexia nervosa. *Pediatric Resident*, 25, 7A.

Kreipe, R. E., Churchill, B. H., & Strauss, J. (1989). Long-term outcome of adolescents with anorexia nervosa. *American Journal of Diseases of Children*, 43, 1322–1327.

Kreipe, R. E., & Harris, J. P. (1993). Myocardial impairment resulting from eating disorders. *Pediatric Annals*, 21, 760–768.

Kreipe, R. E., & Uphoff, M. (1992). Treatment and outcome of adolescents with anorexia nervosa. *Adolescent Medicine: State of the Art Review*, 3, 519–540.

Lanzi, G., Balottin, U., & Borgatti, R. (1987). Follow-up study of thirty-three hospitalized anorectic patients. *International Journal of Psychosomatics*, 34(3), 3–6.

Larson, B. J. (1991). Relationship of family communication patterns to eating disorder inventory scores in adolescent girls. *Journal of American Dietetic Association*, 91, 1065–1067.

Lasègue, E. C. (1873). On hysterical anorexia. In M. R. Kaufman & M. Heiman (Eds.), *Evolution of psychosomatic concepts: Anorexia nervosa—A paradigm* (pp. 298–319). New York: International Universities Press.

Lask, B., & Bryant-Waugh, R. (1992). Early-onset anorexia nervosa and related eating disorders. *Journal of Child Psychology and Psychiatry and Allied Disciplines*, 33, 281–300.

Le Grange, D. (1993). Family therapy outcome in adolescent anorexia nervosa. *South African Journal of Psychology*, 23(4), 174–179.

Le Grange, D. (2005). Family assessment. In J. E. Mitchell & C. B. Peterson (Eds.), *Assessment of eating disorders* (pp. 150–174). New York: Guilford Press.

Le Grange, D., Binford, R., & Loeb, K. L. (2005). Manualized family-based treatment for anorexia nervosa: A case series. *Journal of the American Academy of Child and Adolescent Psychiatry, 44*(1), 41–46.

Le Grange, D., Eisler, I., Dare, C., & Hodes, M. (1992). Family criticism and self-starvation: A study of expressed emotion. *Journal of Family Therapy, 14,* 177–192.

Le Grange, D., Eisler, I., Dare, C., & Russell, G. F. M. (1992). Evaluation of family treatments in adolescent anorexia nervosa: A pilot study. *International Journal of Eating Disorders, 12*(4), 347–357.

Le Grange, D., Lock, J., & Dymek, M. (2003). Family-based therapy for adolescents with bulimia nervosa. *American Journal of Psychotherapy, 67,* 237–251.

Le Grange, D., Loeb, K., Van Orman, S., & Jellar, C. (2004). Adolescent bulimia nervosa: A disorder in evolution? *Archives of Pediatrics and Adolescent Medicine, 158,* 478–482.

Le Grange, D., Crosby, R., Rathauz, P., & Leventhal, B. (2006). *A controlled comparison of family-based treatment and individual supportive psychotherapy for adolescents with bulimia.* Manuscript submitted for publication.

Le Grange, D., & Schmidt, U. (2005). The treatment of adolescents with bulimia nervosa. *Journal of Mental Health, 14*(6), 587–597.

Leon, G. R., Fulkerson, J. A., Perry, C. L., & Cudeck, R. (1992). Personality and behavioral vulnerabilities associated with risk status for eating disorders in adolescent girls. *Journal of Abnormal Psychology, 102*(3), 438–444.

Liebman, R., Minuchin, S., & Baker, L. (1974). An integrated treatment program of anorexia nervosa. *American Journal of Psychiatry, 131,* 432–436.

Liebman, R., Sargent, J., & Silver, M. (1983). A family systems approach to the treatment of anorexia nervosa. *Journal of the American Academy of Child Psychiatry, 22,* 128–133.

Lock, J., Agras, W. S., Bryson, S., & Kraemer, H. C. (2005). A comparison of short- and long-term family therapy for adolescent anorexia nervosa. *Journal of the American Academy of Child and Adolescent Psychiatry, 44*(7), 632–639.

Lock, J., & Le Grange, D. (2005). *Help your teenager beat an eating disorder.* New York: Guilford Press.

Lock, J., Le Grange, D., Agras, W. S., & Dare, C. (2001). *Treatment manual for anorexia nervosa: A family-based approach.* New York: Guilford Press.

Lucas, A. R., Beard, C. M., O'Fallon, W. M., & Kurland, L. T. (1991). 50-year trends in the incidence of anorexia nervosa in Rochester, Minnesota: A population-based study. *American Journal of Psychiatry, 148,* 917–922.

Madanes, C. (1981). *Strategic family therapy.* San Francisco: Jossey-Bass.

Maddocks, S. E., Kaplan, A. S., Woodside, D. B., Langdon, L., & Piran, N. (1992). Two year follow-up of bulimia nervosa: The importance of abstinence as the criterion of outcome. *International Journal of Eating Disorders, 12,* 133–141.

Maloney, M., McGuire, J., & Daniels, S. (1988). Reliability testing of a children's version of the Eating Attitudes Test. *Journal of the American Academy of Child and Adolescent Psychiatry, 27,* 541–543.

McKenzie, J. M. (1992). Hospitalization for anorexia nervosa. *International Journal of Eating Disorders, 11*(3), 235–241.

Minuchin, S., Baker, L., Rosman, B. L., Liebman, R., Milman, L., & Todd, T. C. (1975). A conceptual model of psychosomatic illness in children. *Archives of General Psychiatry, 32,* 1031–1038.

Minuchin, S., Rosman, B. L., & Baker, B. L. (1978). *Psychosomatic families: Anorexia nervosa in context.* Cambridge, MA: Harvard University Press.

Mitchell, J. E., Hatsukami, D., Pyle, R. L., & Eckert, E. D. (1987). Late onset bulimia. *Comprehensive Psychiatry, 28*(4), 323–328.

Morgan, H. G., & Hayward, A. E. (1988). Clinical assessment of anorexia nervosa: The Morgan–Russell Outcome Assessment Schedule. *British Journal of Psychiatry, 152,* 367–371.

Morgan, H. G., & Russell, G. F. M. (1975). Value of family background and clinical features as predictors of long-term outcome in anorexia nervosa: A four year follow-up study of 41 patients. *Psychological Medicine, 5,* 355–371.

Nozoe, S., Soejima, Y., Yoshioka, M., Naruo, T., Masuda, A., Nagai, N., et al. (1995). Clinical features of patients with anorexia nervosa: Assessment of factors influencing the duration of inpatient treatment. *Journal of Psychosomatic Research, 39*(3), 271–281.

Palla, B., & Litt, I. F. (1988). Medical complications of eating disorders in adolescents. *Pediatrics, 81,* 613–623.

Palmer, E. P., & Guay, A. T. (1985). Reversible myopathy secondary to abuse of ipecac in patients with major eating disorders. *New England Journal of Medicine, 313,* 1457–1459.

Palmer, R., Oppenheimer, R., Dignon, A., Chalnor, D., & Howells, K. (1990). Childhood sexual experiences with adults reported by women with eating disorders: An extended series. *British Journal of Psychiatry, 156,* 699–703.

Patton, G. (1988). Mortality in eating disorders. *Psychological Medicine, 18,* 947–961.

Pomeroy, C., Mitchell, J. E., & Eckert, E. D. (1992). Risk of infection and immune function in anorexia nervosa. *International Journal of Eating Disorders, 12,* 47–55.

Pumariega, A. (1986). Acculturation and eating attitudes in adolescent girls: A comparative and correlational study. *Journal of the American Academy of Child and Adolescent Psychiatry, 25*(2), 276–279.

Radke-Sharpe, N., Whitney-Saltiel, D., & Rodin, J. (1990). Fat distribution as a risk factor for weight and eating concerns. *International Journal of Eating Disorders, 9*(1), 27–36.

Rastam, M. (1992). AN in 51 Swedish adolescents: Premorbid problems and comorbidity. *Journal of the American Academy of Child and Adolescent Psychiatry, 31,* 819–828.

Ratnasuriya, R. H., Eisler, I., & Szmukler, G. I. (1991). Anorexia nervosa: Outcome and prognostic factors after 20 years. *British Journal of Psychiatry, 158,* 495–502.

Roberto, L. G. (1986). Bulimia: The transgenerational view. *Journal of Marital and Family Therapy, 12,* 231–240.

Robin, A. L., Siegel, P. T., Koepke, T., Moye, A. W., & Tice, S. (1994). Family therapy versus individual therapy for adolescent females with anorexia nervosa. *Journal of Developmental and Behavioral Pediatrics, 15*(2), 111–116.

Robin, A. L., Seigel, P. T., Moye, A. W., Gilroy, M., Dennis, A. B., & Sikand, A. (1999). A controlled comparison of family versus individual therapy for adolescents with anorexia nervosa. *Journal of the American Academy of Child and Adolescent Psychiatry, 38*(12), 1428–1489.

Root, M. P. P., Fallon, P., & Friedrich, W. N. (1986). *Bulimia: A systems approach to treatment.* New York: Norton.

Rorty, M., Yager, J., & Rossotto, E. (1994). Childhood sexual, physical, and psychological abuse in bulimia nervosa. *American Journal of Psychiatry, 151,* 1122–1126.

Rosman, B. L., Minuchin, S., & Liebman, R. (1975). Family lunch session: An introduction to family therapy for anorexia nervosa. *American Journal of Orthopsychiatry, 45,* 846–853.

Russell, G. F. M. (1979). Bulimia nervosa: An ominous variant of anorexia nervosa. *Psychological Medicine, 9,* 429–448.

Russell, G. F. M. (1992). Anorexia nervosa of early onset and its impact on puberty. In P. F. Cooper & A. Stein (Eds.), *Monographs in clinical pediatrics: Vol. 5. Feeding problems and eating disorders in children and adolescents* (pp. 85–113). Warsaw, Poland: Harwood Academic.

Russell, G. F. M., Szmukler, G. I., Dare, C., & Eisler, I. (1987). An evaluation of family therapy in anorexia nervosa and bulimia nervosa. *Archives of General Psychiatry, 44,* 1047–1056.

Rutherford, J., McGuffin, P., Kutz, R. J., & Murray, R. M. (1993). Genetic influences on eating attitudes in a normal female twin population. *Psychological Medicine, 23,* 425–436.

Schebendach, J., & Nussbaum, M. P. (1992). Nutrition management in adolescents with eating disorders. *Adolescent Medicine State of the Art Reviews, 3,* 541–548.

Schwartz, R. C., Barrett, M. J., & Saba, G. (1985). Family therapy for bulimia. In D. M. Garner & P. E. Garfinkel (Eds.), *Handbook of psychotherapy for anorexia nervosa and bulimia* (pp. 280–307). New York: Guilford Press.

Selvini Palazzoli, M. (1974). *Self-starvation: From the intrapsychic to the transpersonal approach.* London: Chaucer.

Sharpe, T., Ryst, E., Hinshaw, S., & Steiner, H. (1998). Reports of stress: A comparison between eating disorders and normal adolescents. *Child Psychiatry and Child Development, 28,* 117–132.

Shaw, E., Ryst, E., & Steiner, H. (1997). Temperament in juvenile eating disorders. *Psychosomatics, 38,* 126–131.

Shore, R. A., & Porter, J. E. (1990). Normative and reliability data for 11 to 18 year olds on the Eating Disorder Inventory. *International Journal of Eating Disorders, 9*(2), 201–207.

Silber, T. J., Delaney, D., & Samuels, J. (1989). Anorexia nervosa: Hospitalization in adolescent medicine units and third-party payments. *Journal of Adolescent Health Care, 10,* 122–125.

Smith, C., Nasserbakht, A., Feldman, S., & Steiner, H. (1993). Psychological characteristics and DSM-III-R diagnoses at six-year follow-up of adolescent anorexia nervosa. *Journal of American Academy of Child and Adolescent Psychiatry, 32*(6), 1237–1245.

Society for Adolescent Medicine. (1995). Eating disorders in adolescents: A position paper of the Society for Adolescent Medicine. *Journal of Adolescent Health, 16,* 476–480.

Steiger, H., Leung, F., & Houle, L. (1992). Relationships among borderline features, body dissatisfactions and bulimic symptoms in nonclinical families. *Addictive Behaviors, 17*(4), 397–406.

Stein, S., Chalhoub, N., & Hodes, M. (1998). Very early onset bulimia nervosa: Report of two cases. *International Journal of Eating Disorders, 24,* 323–327.

Steiner, H., & Lock, J. (1998). Eating disorders in children and adolescents: A review of the past ten years. *Journal of the American Academy of Child and Adolescent Psychiatry*, 37(4), 352–359.

Steiner, H., Lock, J., & Reissel, B. (1999). Developmental approaches to diagnosis and treatment of eating disorders. *La Revue Prisme*, 52–67.

Steiner, H., Mazer, C., & Litt, I. (1990). Compliance and outcome in AN. *Western Journal of Medicine*, 153, 133–139.

Steiner, H., Sanders, M., & Ryst, E. (1995). Precursors and risk factors of juvenile eating disorders. In H. D. Steinhausen (Ed.), *Eating disorders in adolescence: Anorexia and bulimia nervosa* (pp. 95–125). New York: de Gruyter.

Steiner, H., Smith, C., Rosenkrantz, R., & Litt, I. F. (1991). The early care and feeding of anorexics. *Child Psychiatry and Human Development*, 21(3), 163–167.

Steinhausen, H. C. (Ed.). (1995). *Eating disorders in adolescence*. New York: de Gruyter.

Steinhausen, H. C., Rauss-Mason, C., & Seidel, R. (1991). Follow-up studies of anorexia nervosa: A review of four decades of outcome research. *Psychological Medicine*, 21, 447–454.

Steinhausen, H. C., Rauss-Mason, C., & Seidel, R. (1993). Short-term and intermediate term outcome in adolescent eating disorders. *Acta Psychiatrica Scandinavica*, 88, 169–173.

Stevens, J., Story, M., Ring, K., Murray, D. M., Cornell, C. E., Juhaeri, J., & Gittelsohn, J. (2003). The impact of the Pathways intervention on psychosocial variables related to diet and physical activity in American Indian schoolchildren. *Preventive Medicine: An International Journal Devoted to Practice and Theory*, 37(6, Pt. 2), S70–S79.

Stice, E., Agras, S., & Hammer, L. (1999). Risk factors for the emergence of childhood eating disturbances: A five-year prospective study. *International Journal of Eating Disorders*, 25, 375–387.

Stice, E., Killen, J. D., Hayward, C., & Taylor, C. B. (1998). Age of onset for binge eating and purging during late adolescence: A 4-year survival analysis. *Journal of Abnormal Psychology*, 107(4), 671–675.

Story, M., French, S. A., Resnick, M. D., & Blum, R. W. (1995). Ethnic/racial and socioeconomic differences in dieting behaviors and body image perceptions in adolescents. *International Journal of Eating Disorders*, 18(2), 173–179.

Strober, H. (1990). Family-genetic studies of eating disorders. *Journal of Clinical Psychiatry*, 52(10), 9–12.

Strober, M. (1991). Disorders of the self in anorexia nervosa: An organismic–developmental paradigm. In C. Johnson (Ed.), *Psychodynamic treatment of anorexia nervosa and bulimia* (pp. 354–373). New York: Guilford Press.

Szmukler, G., Eisler, I., Russell, G., & Dare, C. (1985). Anorexia nervosa: Parental "expressed emotion" and dropping out of treatment. *British Journal of Psychiatry*, 147, 265–271.

Toner, D. D., Garfinkel, P. E., & Garner, D. M. (1986). Long-term follow-up of anorexia nervosa. *Psychosomatic Medicine*, 48, 320–329.

Treasure, L., Todd, G., Brolly, M., Tiller, J., Nehmed, A., & Denman, F. (1995). A pilot study of a randomized trial of cognitive analytical therapy vs educational behavioral therapy for adult anorexia nervosa. *Behaviour Research and Therapy*, 33(4), 363–367.

Van der-ham, T., van Strien, D. C., & van England, H. (1994). A four-year prospective follow-up of 49 eating disorder adolescents: Differences in course of illness. *Acta Psychiatrica Scandinavica*, 90(3), 229–235.

Vaughn, C., & Leff, J. (1976). The influence of family and social factors on the course of psychiatric illness: A comparison of schizophrenic and depressed neurotic patients. *British Journal of Psychiatry, 129*, 125–137.

Walford, G., & McCune, W. (1991). Long-term outcome in early-onset anorexia nervosa. *British Journal of Psychiatry, 159*, 383–389.

Waller, G. (1991). Sexual abuse as a factor in eating disorders. *British Journal of Psychiatry, 159*, 664–671.

Walsh, B. T., & Wilson, G. T. (1997). *Supportive psychotherapy manual. Appendix II, bulimia nervosa treatment trial.* Unpublished manual, Columbia University, New York, NY, and Rutgers University, Piscataway, NJ.

Webster, J. J., & Palmer, R. L. (2000). The childhood and family background of women with clinical eating disorders: A comparison with women with major depression and women without psychiatric disorder. *Psychological Medicine, 30*, 53–60.

Whitaker, A., Johnson, J., Shaffer, D., Rapoport, J. L., Kalikow, K., Walsh, B. T., et al. (1990). Uncommon troubles in young people: Prevalence estimates of selected psychiatric disorders in a nonreferred adolescent population. *Archives of General Psychiatry, 47*, 487–496.

Windauer, U., Lennerts, W., Talbot, P., Touyz, S. W., & Beumont, P. J. (1993). How will one "cure" anorexia nervosa patients? An investigation of 16 weight-recovered anorectic patients. *British Journal of Psychiatry, 163*, 195–200.

Wynne, L. C. (1980). Paradoxical interventions: Leverage for therapeutic change in individual and family systems. In M. Strauss, T. Bowers, S. Downey, S. Fleck, & I. Levin (Eds.), *The psychotherapy of schizophrenia* (pp. 191–202). New York: Plenum Press.

Yager, J., Andersen, A., Devlin, M., Mitchell, J., Powers, P., & Yates, A. (1993). American Psychiatric Association practice guidelines for eating disorders. *American Journal of Psychiatry, 150*, 207–228.

Yates, A. (1990). Current perspectives on the eating disorders: II. Treatment, outcome, and research directions. *Journal of the American Academy of Child and Adolescent Psychiatry, 29*, 1–9.

Zipfel, S., Löwe, B., & Herzog, W. (2005). Medical complications. In J. Treasure, U. Schmidt, & E. van Furth (Eds.), *The essential handbook of eating disorders* (pp. 53–74). Chichester, UK: Wiley.

Index